SpringerBriefs in Well-Being and Quality of Life Research

More information about this series at http://www.springer.com/series/10150

Toni Noble · Helen McGrath

The PROSPER School Pathways for Student Wellbeing

Policy and Practices

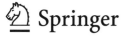 Springer

Toni Noble
Institute for Positive Psychology
    and Education
Australian Catholic University
Strathfield, NSW
Australia

Helen McGrath
School of Education
Deakin University
Burwood, VIC
Australia

ISSN 2211-7644   ISSN 2211-7652 (electronic)
SpringerBriefs in Well-Being and Quality of Life Research
ISBN 978-3-319-21794-9   ISBN 978-3-319-21795-6 (eBook)
DOI 10.1007/978-3-319-21795-6

Library of Congress Control Number: 2015948716

Springer Cham Heidelberg New York Dordrecht London

Springer International Publishing AG Switzerland is part of Springer Science+Business Media
(www.springer.com)

Contents

Chapter 1
Student Skills for Happiness and Wellbeing

Abstract This chapter outlines the key student skills and understandings for happiness and wellbeing at school and in their future, followed by a research-based definition of student wellbeing. The difference between student wellbeing and student welfare is clarified and then evidence-based guidelines are provided to help practitioners select effective student wellbeing programs. The chapter concludes by introducing PROSPER as an organising framework for the components of wellbeing that underpin positive psychological research and can be applied in positive education. The PROSPER components are **P**ositivity, **R**elationships, **O**utcomes, **S**trengths, **P**urpose, **E**ngagement and **R**esilience.

Keywords Student wellbeing · Positive psychology · Positive education · Social-emotional learning programs

1.1 Introduction

One of the most important goals for any country is that its children and young people enjoy their lives and acquire the skills and understandings to become happy, functioning adults. Education has a key role to play in equipping young people with the knowledge, understanding and skills they will need in order to live fulfilling lives and to be productive in the flexible and innovative workforce required in this 21st century. A school-based focus on supporting children and young people to develop a deep sense of wellbeing is a central component of effective education for their future, their country's future and for the future of our world.

1.2 Outline of Chapters

This chapter outlines the key student skills and understandings for happiness and wellbeing at school and in their future, followed by a research-based definition of student wellbeing. The difference between student wellbeing and student welfare is

© The Author(s) 2016
T. Noble and H. McGrath, *The PROSPER School Pathways for Student Wellbeing*,
SpringerBriefs in Well-Being and Quality of Life Research,
DOI 10.1007/978-3-319-21795-6_1

clarified and then evidence-based guidelines are provided to help practitioners select effective student wellbeing programs. This chapter concludes by introducing PROSPER as an organising framework for the components of wellbeing that underpin positive psychological research and can be applied in positive education. Chapter 2 then follows by applying the PROSPER organiser to the evidence-based school practices that can enhance student happiness and wellbeing. Chapter 3 reviews guidelines/actions for developing a student wellbeing policy at the school, system, national and international levels.

1.3   Why Does Student Wellbeing Matter?

About one-third of the world's population is under 18 years of age (UNICEF 2014). In any country (rich or poor) about 10 % or 220 million children and young people have a diagnosable mental disorder (mainly anxiety, depression or conduct disorder) (WHO 2003; Global Burden of Disease Study 2010 2012). Over half of the children who experience mental illness in childhood will also suffer from a mental illness in their adult lives (Kim-Cohen et al. 2003; Layard and Hagell 2015) which means their lives are likely to be unhappy and impoverished. Mental health also affects physical health. In the richest countries only 25 % of children with mental health issues receive specialist help and in the poorest countries very few have access to any help (Layard and Hagell 2015). From humanitarian perspective this is a great loss but it also comes at an economic cost. In most countries mental illness is reducing gross domestic product (GDP) by over 5 % (OECD 2014). Wellbeing is a set of skills that can be taught. The aim of all countries is for their children to be educated at school. So a core concern for all schools around the world needs to be how can they best develop their student's sense of wellbeing, not just their academic performance so they can thrive and prosper.

1.4   C21st Skills and Understandings for Student Wellbeing

A focus on student wellbeing is integral to the United Nations goals for education that are to make people wiser, more knowledgeable, better informed, ethical, responsible citizens who are critical thinkers, and capable of and motivated to become life-long learners. At the beginning of the 21st century the United Nations adopted four pillars for student wellbeing. These four pillars are learning to live together, learning to know, learning to do and learning to be (Delors 1996). Here we describe and build on each pillar to provide a useful frame of reference for the essential skills and understandings that enable students to flourish firstly at school and then later in the workplace and in their life in the 21st century.

1. Pillar One: Learning to LIVE TOGETHER
   This Pillar highlights the importance of explicitly teaching young people the values and social-emotional competencies that connect people, build relationships, strengthen communities and enhance their valuing of social, cultural and religious diversity. This pillar also recognises the critical interdependence of a young person's local community with our global community and the importance of developing their skills to be able to work collaboratively with others both locally and globally to achieve mutual goals. This pillar extends to developing students as active and informed citizens who act with moral and ethical integrity and develop into responsible local and global citizens.
2. Pillar Two: Learning to KNOW
   This pillar identifies the importance of helping young people to '*learn how to learn*' along with the more traditional focus on the acquisition of structured discipline knowledge. Learning '*how to learn*' refers to developing students' skills in using effective thinking skills such as the capacity for critical and creative thinking, using evidence in support of propositions and initiatives, solving problems both analytically and ethically and making evidence-informed decisions. These skills enable students to adapt to change and to be critical and creative in finding new solutions to diverse and complex problems.
3. Pillar Three: Learning to DO
   The focus of this pillar is on the importance of supporting young people to develop capabilities in the diverse range of general work-related skills required for work success, whatever their chosen occupation. These capabilities include good communication skills, teamwork and collaborative skills and problem solving skills as well as the capacity to cope resiliently in difficult and challenging situations or in times of adversity.
4. Pillar Four: Learning to BE
   The emphasis in this pillar is on the importance of stimulating the imagination and creativity of young people through the provision of opportunities and encouragement to undertake aesthetic, artistic, scientific, cultural and social discoveries and to develop their confidence in experimentation.

These four pillars align with the outcomes from a recent major international project that involved a group of 250 researchers across 60 institutions worldwide (Griffin et al. 2012). Ten key skills for learners evolved from an analysis of international educational curricula and assessment frameworks. These ten skills fall into four broad categories:

1. **Ways of thinking** (*learning to know*)

   (a) Creativity and innovation
   (b) Critical thinking, problem-solving and decision-making
   (c) Learning to learn and metacognition

2. **Ways of working** (*learning to do*)

   (a) Communication
   (b) Collaboration and teamwork

3. **Tools for working**

   (a) Information and communications technology (ICT)
   (b) Information literacy (includes research on sources, evidence, biases, etc.)

4. **Skills for living in the world** (*learning to live together*)

   (a) Citizenship-local and global
   (b) Life and career
   (c) Personal and social responsibility (including cultural awareness and competence).

These ten skills identified by Griffin et al. (2012) and the four pillars identified by the United Nations (Delors 1996) represent life skills, not skills that are mainly learned at school and relevant only to academic learning. One key difference between the two frameworks is the focus in the more recent study by Griffin et al. (2012) on the importance of young people becoming life-long learners of skills related to the use of ever-changing information and communications technologies. These skills have become increasingly important over the last 15 years in Western countries as well as in developing countries, with widespread mobile phone networks now available globally. A focus on skills related to information and communication technologies recognises that learning and working in the 21st century can occur at any time and any place, not just in schools or workplaces.

In 2013 the first author was invited by the King and Government of Bhutan to attend an International Expert Meeting in Thimpu co-sponsored by the United Nations. The goal of the meeting was to develop a new global model for happiness and wellbeing 'a new development paradigm'. The international team included participants from UK, Europe, USA, South America and Australia. Bhutan's focus on happiness and wellbeing began over thirty years ago when the fourth king of Bhutan famously proclaimed that gross national happiness is more important than gross national productivity. Following this historic declaration, Bhutan developed a Gross National Happiness (GNH) Index and screening tool to evaluate all their new policies. This index evaluates nine domains of happiness: education, psychological wellbeing, community vitality, time use, health, living standards, cultural diversity, good governance and ecological diversity The education domain is central to all nine domains of GNH. Education is intrinsically dynamic and transformative. Thus education serves as the key thread that connects all nine domains of GNH and offers the most leverage for individual, local and global happiness and wellbeing.

One of the key recommendations that emerged from this meeting in Bhutan was that the older concept of '*skills for living in the world/living together*' should be extended to focus on the roots of deep abiding happiness that comes from living life in full harmony with the natural world, with our own communities and fellow beings, and with our culture and spiritual heritage (New Development Paradigm).

The implication for schools is that identifying and implementing strategies for enhancing student happiness and wellbeing at school should become a major component of the work of teachers and schools.

In recent times school systems, governments and policy makers around the world are increasingly focusing on the role of coordinated school-based student wellbeing initiatives. Many researchers have identified the inter-dependence of student wellbeing and student learning (Zins et al. 2004; Durlak et al. 2011).

1.5 Defining Student Wellbeing

A logical starting point for educating for student wellbeing is to work from a robust and evidence-based definition of student wellbeing that has the power to effectively guide educational policy and school practices. Naturally a child's family, home and community all significantly impact on a young person's wellbeing. However an educational perspective focuses on the actions that schools and school systems can adopt to help children and young people flourish within a school context.

Although there are many definitions of wellbeing, a literature search revealed only three definitions of *student wellbeing* (Noble et al. 2008). One definition identified student wellbeing as:

> a positive emotional state that is the result of a harmony between the sum of specific context factors on the one hand and the personal needs and expectations towards the school on the other hand (Engels et al. 2004, p. 128)

Another simpler definition of student wellbeing was:

> the degree to which a student feels good in the school environment (De Fraine et al. 2005)

The third definition focused on student well being as:

> the degree to which a student is functioning effectively in the school community (Fraillon 2004).

A more comprehensive definition of student wellbeing was sought that incorporated multiple dimensions. Noble et al. (2008) used a modified Delphi methodology to develop a robust and operational definition of student wellbeing. The first step was the generation of a broad definition of student wellbeing that integrated selected components from a range of definitions of general wellbeing plus the three definitions of student wellbeing cited above. The second step involved seeking the online involvement of thirty international experts who worked in the field of wellbeing and/or student wellbeing from a range of countries including Australia, Denmark, United Kingdom, Italy, New Zealand, Portugal and the USA. These participants were invited to give feedback on the definition. Their feedback assisted with the re-development of the definition. They were then asked to give feedback on a second amended definition. This process was repeated another two times until a strong degree of agreement was reached on the best definition which is:

> Optimal student wellbeing is a sustainable emotional state characterised by (predominantly) positive mood and attitude, positive relationships with other students and teachers, resilience, self-optimisation, and a high level of satisfaction with their learning experiences at school (Noble et al. 2008; NSSF 2011)

- The term '*optimal student wellbeing*' was used to highlight the 'desirable' level of wellbeing that was most likely to lead to a range of positive student outcomes. The inclusion of the term '*sustainable state*' reflected that wellbeing is a relatively consistent mental or emotional condition that is maintained across time and most school-based contexts
- '*Predominantly positive mood, attitude and relationships at school*' highlights that students with optimal wellbeing experience mainly positive feelings about being at school and that their relationships with peers and teachers engenders a sense of social satisfaction and support.
- The term '*resilience*' refers to the importance of a student having enough skills and support to 'bounce back' emotionally when things don't go well at school. Nearly all definitions of resilience refer to the capacity of the individual to demonstrate the personal strengths that are needed to cope with challenges, difficulties, hardship, challenge or adversity. Resilience has been defined as '*the ability to persist, cope adaptively and bounce back after encountering change, challenges, setback, disappointments, difficult situations or adversity and to return to a reasonable level of wellbeing*' (McGrath and Noble 2003, 2011). It is also the *capacity to respond adaptively to difficult circumstances and still thrive* (McGrath and Noble 2011).
- '*Self-optimisation*' means having a realistic awareness of one's own strengths, abilities and skills and demonstrating a willingness to use this self knowledge to maximise their perceived potential in many areas (e.g. intellectual, social, emotional, physical and spiritual).
- '*A high level of satisfaction with learning experiences at school*' describes a student's satisfaction with the quality and relevance of their learning experiences at school and their own level of involvement in these learning experiences.

Ryan and Deci (2001) have described the field of wellbeing research as falling into two camps: that which focuses on hedonism (pleasure) and that which focuses on eudaimonism (fulfillment via actualisation of one's potential). This definition of student wellbeing integrates:

(i) the subjective (or hedonic) construct of wellbeing that encompasses how students evaluate their life at school; the affective component (how they feel), and the cognitive component (their perceptions and thoughts about their life at school) and

(ii) the eudaimonic construct of wellbeing, in which wellbeing is construed as an ongoing and positive dynamic process rather than a fixed state through the notion of self-optimisation or students' fulfilling their potential.

The construct of 'abiding happiness' (as proposed in Bhutan's New Development Paradigm 2013) goes further than the hedonic and eudaimonic constructs of wellbeing and explicitly includes concern for others, for one's community and culture and for the natural environment. To further the goal of abiding happiness it is recommended that educational policies to promote student wellbeing integrate all of the above constructs. Research indicates that a student with an optimal level of wellbeing is more likely to have higher levels of school attendance, demonstrate age-appropriate academic skills, engage in more pro-social behaviour and be less likely to bully others (Noble et al. 2008; Durlak et al. 2011).

1.5.1 Student Wellbeing Is not the Same as Student Welfare

There is some confusion in the research literature between the concepts of 'student welfare' and 'student wellbeing' within a school context. 'Student welfare' refers to an approach in which a qualified professional such as a psychologist, social worker or social welfare worker identifies students in need of assistance, comfort or support as a result of their experiences of adverse, disabling or distressing circumstances. These circumstances may be (for example) financial, social, physical, cultural, familial and/or psychological. They then select the appropriate actions from a diverse range of options. A student welfare approach is more of a reactive approach to identified concerns with students rather than a proactive approach adopted by a student wellbeing focus. In contrast to student welfare, a focus on student wellbeing reviews the school policies, structures and activities that contribute to students 'feeling good and functioning well' at school and building schools as enabling institutions.

1.6 What Is a Student Wellbeing Program?

A student wellbeing program is a planned and coordinated program of content, activities and strategies that focuses on creating a positive learning environment and teaching students the values, attitudes and skills that have the power to enhance their quality of life, their relationships, their connectedness to school and their learning and achievement.

1.6.1 Guidelines for Choosing Implementing and Sustaining Student Wellbeing Programs

The available research evidence strongly indicates the following guidelines for the effective implementation and sustainability of social and emotional learning programs in schools. See Chap. 3 page 100 for five stages of Quality Implementation Programs Based on Social-Emotional Learning.

1.6.1.1 Universal Programs Have More Impact

A universal program is presented to all students, not just to those who have been identified as being at risk for mental health and/or behavioural difficulties. The aim of universal programs is to develop students' social, emotional and behavioural competencies. The belief is that all students can benefit from learning the targeted skills such as social skills, coping skills and problem-solving skills (Durlak et al. 2011; Greenberg et al. 2001). Universal programs focus on primary prevention and include classroom-based approaches as well as changes to the school environment and may also include family and community. According to the World Health Organisation's health promotion model, the greatest amount of time and resources should be spent on universal approaches that include the whole school.

However selected and targeted interventions have also been found as important for students at risk (selected) or identified with behavioural, emotional or mental health problem. Here the focus is on additional individualised learning sessions (Sugai et al. 2009).

1.6.1.2 Whole-School Programs Can Contribute to a Positive School Culture

A whole school program means all classes are taught the program at developmentally appropriate levels. In contrast most programs target one whole age cohort in a school, and produce good results in the short term but these results are usually not sustained. This is not surprising given that the programs typically average 20 h (Durlak et al. 2011). A whole school program presented for one hour a week throughout a student's school life provides important opportunities for the key skills and understandings to be learned in age-appropriate ways and the repetition ensures a greater opportunity for deep 'habitual' learning (Layard and Hagell 2015; McGrath and Noble 2011).

A whole school program also means that it is easier to communicate the key messages to the students' families and the school community through school newsletters, assembly items, school concerts and performances etc. (Noble and McGrath 2014; Greenberg et al. 2003). A whole-school program is also more effective in developing a positive school culture rather than an 'add-on' program (Noble and McGrath 2014; Axford et al. 2011; Wells et al. 2003). A positive school culture has been shown to be significantly related to improved outcomes for students such as stronger motivation to achieve and better academic results, increased pro-social behaviour, and higher school connectedness (O'Malley et al. 2012). A positive school culture also impacts on teacher outcomes such as higher levels of teacher efficacy and greater work satisfaction (O'Malley et al. 2012).

1.6.1.3   Strong Leadership Support Is Crucial

Instrumental to successful implementation and sustainability of a program is the support of the school leadership team for the program. This support provided by the principal and ideally a student wellbeing coordinator (or a staff member in a similar role), can be in terms of timing (when), resources, incentives and professional development. Leadership support can also determine the intensity of the program implementation (how often and in what form) and the duration (for how long) of the intervention (Shonkoff and Phillips 2000). Leadership support helps to make a program a school priority and to sustain its implementation (Noble and McGrath 2014; Han and Weiss 2005; Kam et al. 2003). This support also means that the program is more likely to be directly aligned to a school's improvement plan, school values and school, classroom and playground practices. In this way a consistent message is communicated to the whole school community.

Leadership support can also be instrumental in achieving effective implementation of a program by ensuring a reasonable balance between a school's fidelity to the program and adaptation (Durlak 2015). Fidelity refers to delivering the core components of the program that power the intervention. Adaptations make the program a 'good fit' for their school.

1.6.1.4   School System/District Support

Linking the program's objectives not only to the school's vision and priorities but also to the mission and priorities of the school district, state and/or national priority provides more support to the school leadership team to sustain the program's implementation over years (Noble and McGrath 2014; Adelman and Taylor 2003; Elias et al. 2003). For example at the system level the Catholic Education Office in Melbourne have funded over 1000 teachers to complete a Masters degree in Student Wellbeing and supported schools to embed social-emotional learning in their curriculum. Another example at the National level is the Australian Government's KidsMatter (primary) and MindMatter (secondary) mental health initiatives that provide support to schools to choose and implement a whole school social-emotional learning program.

1.6.1.5   Programs that Are Taught by Class Teachers and Integrated with Academic Learning Are More Likely to Be Effective

Academic improvement as well as social and emotional improvement is more likely when teachers (rather than external consultants or professionals) implement a social-emotional learning program (Durlak et al. 2011; Weissberg and O'Brien 2004). Based on their knowledge of their students' needs, the classroom teacher is also able to provide targeted support; for example choosing to teach resilience skills to the whole class which benefits everyone but particularly a couple of highly anxious students. Teachers are also able to utilise 'teachable moments' (e.g. after a bullying incident) that can provide a 'real world' opportunity to teach or reinforce the relevant skills and values to encourage the students to immediately apply these skills in context (Noble and McGrath 2014).

1.6.1.6 The Program Needs to Be Acceptable to Teachers

Teachers are more motivated to effectively implement and sustain programs that they perceive to be acceptable (Elias et al. 2003; Han and Weiss 2005; Eckert and Hintz 2000); feasible, worth their time and effort and socially valid (Barry et al. 2013; Han and Weiss 2005; Gresham and Lopez 1996). Such programs are those that reflect their knowledge and values and are consistent with their educational, psychological and social perspectives and classroom practices. Teachers also need to perceive that they have the necessary competencies to teach the program (Bandura 1996). The program should also have some degree of flexibility so it can be adapted and customised to meet the needs of their school and students (Han and Weiss 2005). One of the most significant factors that contribute to a program's acceptability in the view of teachers is that the teachers perceive that their students are behaving and learning better as a result of their implementation of the program (Han and Weiss 2005; Datnow and Castellano 2000).

1.6.1.7 Programs that Involve Parents and School Support Staff Are More Likely to Be Effective and Enduring

Programs that involve partnerships with parents and school support staff are more likely to be sustained over time than programs without that partnership (Webster-Stratton and Taylor 2001). School support staff such as counselors and social workers have an important role to play in both enhancing the implementation of a program and reinforcing key knowledge and skills from the program when working with targeted individual students or groups.

Family-school partnerships are more than just parental involvement. They are child-focused approaches in which families and school-based professionals collaborate to provide opportunities for the enhancement of social, emotional and academic outcomes for young people (Kim et al. 2012; Albright and Weissberg 2010). Albright et al. (2011) have recommended the creation of a committee of staff and parents that can focus specifically on communicating, planning and decision-making that will also encourage the involvement of parents in the implementation of programs to support their children's social and emotional learning. Such a committee might include, for example, a senior member of staff such as an assistant principal, the school counsellor and several parents. Some specific strategies that have been suggested by Albright et al. (2011) as contributing to successful school-family partnerships include:

- Creating a family room where parents can meet and chat and which also includes a resource centre where they can choose information sheets or borrow books.
- Highlighting a specific book each month that focuses on an aspect of SEL.
- Asking parents about their preferences for when parent information sessions should be scheduled and which form of home-school communication they prefer (e.g. email, phone or newsletter).
- The use of an online newsletter that highlights specific examples of positive social and emotional behaviours observed by the teachers.
- Involving children in the preparation and decoration of newsletters or invitations to parent information/discussion sessions.

1.6.1.8 Programs that Are Long-Term and Multi-year Have More Chance of Success

Preventive interventions over one or two school terms produce short-term benefits. Multi-year programs where the key messages can be revisited in age-appropriate ways are more likely to produce enduring benefits and are more sustainable especially when taught across age levels (Greenberg et al. 2001, 2003; Wells et al. 2003; Browne et al. 2004).

1.6.1.9 A Multi-strategic and Multi-component Approach Is More Effective Than a Single Highly-Focused Approach

A multi-strategic approach that focuses on the whole child involves a number of coordinated 'active ingredients' rather than a single focus e.g. just social skills or just time management skills (Durlak et al. 2011; Browne et al. 2004; Greenberg et al. 2001; Resnick et al. 1997). A multi-component approach includes different components such as life skills, social skills, literacy skills and may include a school and community component such as the involvement of families. Effective programs contain at least five different aspects of social and emotional learning (Durlak et al. 2011; Catalano et al. 2003) and focus on both promoting positive behaviour and reducing anti-social behaviour (Catalano et al. 1996).

1.6.1.10 Effectiveness Is Enhanced When Children Are First Introduced to the Program Early in Their Schooling

Research has shown that children by the age of ten years have already developed negative or pessimistic habits of thinking which determines how they respond to new situations (Reivich 2005). Prevention programs that start to teach children the key skills and understandings of happiness and wellbeing from the first years of schooling are therefore more likely to be effective (Barry et al. 2013; Browne et al. 2004; Greenberg et al. 2003; O'Shaughnessy et al. 2003).

There are also advocates for implementing prevention programs for preschool-aged children (e.g. Barrett et al. 2014; Luby 2010). Barrett et al. (2014) propose that early childhood prevention initiatives should include both a universal component in which skills and understandings are taught to all children in a pre-school setting as well as a selective component directed towards children identified as displaying behaviours that place them at risk for later social and emotional difficulties. Early childhood is considered to be a particular sensitive (and perhaps even critical) period of neurological development during which social and emotional skills may be more easily developed (Luby 2010). Barrett et al. (2014) also point out that children are more adaptable and flexible at this age and therefore such interventions are more likely to be successful in promoting effective social and emotional skills in children. In particular, having an early opportunity to learn and practise social skills and empathy increases the likelihood that children will have more successful social interactions with their peers at a younger age and be more likely to develop a positive social image of themselves before they start school. Early childhood prevention programs that enable young children to master skills related to resilience, such as self-management, problem-solving skills and coping skills, before they start school, are also more likely to achieve better learning outcomes when they start school.

1.6.1.11   An Effective Program Includes a Significant Component of Skills Derived from Cognitive Behaviour Approaches (CBT)

CBT is based on the understanding that *how you think affects how you feel* which in turn influences *how you behave*. The key message is that by changing a person's thinking from irrational to rational and more positive thinking they can change their behaviour and be happier. The 'coat-hanger' of the Bounce Back Resilience program is the 10 CBT coping statements that make up the Bounce Back acronym (McGrath and Noble 2011). Martin Seligman's Learned Optimism is also based on CBT (Seligman et al. 1995, 1998). A meta-analysis of research on the Penn Resiliency Program (PRP) based on learned optimism found that in 13 randomised controlled trials the program can prevent symptoms of depression (Gillham et al. 2008). However in the PRP studies sample sizes are relatively small and despite the manualised curriculum, the PRP team recommend trained facilitators rather than classroom teachers.

1.6 What Is a Student Wellbeing Program?

1.6.1.12 The Program Should Incorporate Evidence-Informed Teaching Strategies and Focus on the Explicit Teaching of Skills

Programs that also incorporate evidence-informed teaching strategies are more likely to lead to improved social-emotional learning and academic outcomes (Elias 2003). They can also contribute to higher student engagement and thereby gain greater teacher 'buy-in'. Cooperative learning, for example, has extensive evidence support for improving academic outcomes as well as building positive relationships, class cohesion and social-emotional learning (e.g. Hattie 2009; Johnson et al. 2001; Marzano et al. 2001; Roseth et al. 2008). Also adopting a model that includes a combination of explanation, discussion and the explicit teaching of social and emotional skills and the provision of opportunities to practise these skills is more likely to be effective than just an 'explain and hope' model (e.g. see McGrath and Francey 1991; McGrath and Noble 2011).

1.7 Social and Emotional Learning (SEL)

One of the most common components of a student wellbeing program is the teaching of social and emotional skills. These are skills which can be taught to children and young people to enable them to understand and manage their own emotions, set and achieve positive goals, feel and show empathy for others, establish and maintain positive relationships, and make responsible decisions. CASEL (Collaborative for Academic, Social and Emotional learning-http://www.casel.org) has identified five interrelated clusters of social-emotional competencies. These are:

1. *Self-awareness*—recognising one's emotions and values, and being able to realistically assess one's strengths and limitations.
2. *Self-management*—being able to set and achieve goals, and handling one's own emotions so that they facilitate rather than interfere with relevant tasks.
3. *Social awareness*—showing understanding and empathy for the perspective and feelings of others.
4. *Relationship skills*—establishing and maintaining healthy relationships, working effectively in groups as both leader and team member, and dealing constructively with conflict.
5. *Responsible decision-making and problem solving*—making ethical, constructive choices about personal and social behaviour.

Many of the key social and emotional skills that can be explicitly taught to students are also essential workplace skills. For example social skills such as cooperation, working in a team, active listening and negotiation are skills that enhance learning within a school context will also assist students to be successful in their later workplace lives.

The most effective learning of social and emotional skills occurs when high-quality evidence-informed programs are embedded within safe, caring, well-managed and cooperative classroom environments. They also highlight the importance of explicitly teaching specific social and emotional skills both systematically and developmentally. These social-emotional learning programs have been shown to significantly impact on student attendance, student engagement with learning and students' attachment and commitment to their schools. As a result, student wellbeing initiatives that include a strong focus on teaching social and emotional skills have the potential to reduce barriers to learning by building students' sense of wellbeing and their capacity to learn and their connection to school (Zins et al. 2004; Durlak et al. 2011).

The findings of a large-scale meta-analysis of social and emotional learning programs (Durlak et al. 2011) have confirmed the positive impact of student SEL-based wellbeing programs on learning and achievement. The meta-analysis focused on 213 school-based, universal social-emotional learning programs and involved over 270,000 students from primary-school entry to year 12. Compared to controls, students who participated in social-emotional learning programs showed an 11-percentile-point gain in academic achievement. They also showed significant improvements in social and emotional skills, attitudes and behaviour in the school context. Similarly Diekstra and Gravesteijn (2008) conducted a large world-wide meta-analysis of nineteen earlier meta-analyses (published between 1997 and 2008) evaluating the effectiveness of student wellbeing programs that focused on teaching social and emotional skills. These studies had focused on either primary or secondary schools and comprised many hundreds of thousands of students. Their conclusions were that student wellbeing programs that focused predominantly on social and emotional skills or 'skills for life':

- significantly enhanced students' social and emotional competence,
- significantly reduced or prevented behaviour and mental heath problems or disorders (e.g. *truancy, dropping out of secondary school, aggression, criminal behaviour, misuse of drugs and alcohol and symptoms of mental health difficulties such as anxiety and depression*),
- significantly enhanced or promoted school-connectedness and positive attitudes and behaviours by students towards themselves, others and their school,
- significantly enhanced academic achievement, and
- benefited students from low socio-economic status and different ethnic backgrounds at least as much as other students (and often more).

Diekstra et al. (2008) concluded that enhanced social and emotional development is the key to the overall development of students in terms of their academic progress, school career and societal functioning.

More recently the World Health Organisation commissioned a review of mental health promotion interventions in low and middle income countries (Barry et al. 2013). These countries were Gaza/Palestine, South Africa, Uganda, India, Chile, Mauritius, Nepal, and Lebanon. The majority of the studies (>60 %) were published between 2010–2012. Findings from the 14 school-based interventions indicated reasonably robust evidence that school-based programmes implemented in these diverse countries can have significant positive effects on students' emotional and behavioural wellbeing, including reduced depression and anxiety and improved coping skills. An example of a positive community intervention was a teacher led peer-group support intervention for AIDs orphaned children in a low-income country. This study indicated the potential of peer support mental health promotion interventions in optimizing adjustment and decreasing the psychological distress associated with AIDS orphanhood in the adolescent age group. Given difficulties with sometimes accessing teachers, Barry et al. (2013) concluded that such community interventions engaging peer support may have great potential in low income countries to address the increased risk of depression, peer relationship problems, post-traumatic stress and conduct problems in at risk populations such as AIDS orphans. One identified problem is that almost all the interventions were short-term and limited in their scope in terms of the number of students with access to the intervention. The review recommends that the interventions are expanded to regional and national levels and inform educational and health national policies.

Two examples of a National initiative that impacts on education and health is Australia's KidsMatter and MindMatter frameworks. KidsMatter and MindMatter are flexible Australian student mental health and wellbeing framework funded by the Australian Government and backed by the expertise of the Australian Psychological Society, Beyondblue, Early Childhood Australia and the Principals Australia Institute. The purpose is to assist primary schools, pre-schools and care centres (KidsMatter) and secondary schools (MindMatter) to enhance the mental health and wellbeing of their students/children by creating settings and conducting programs that support students' social and emotional wellbeing needs. KidsMatter provides an online directory of student wellbeing programs that describes each program and indicates whether or not they have been evaluated. An evaluation of 100 schools who participated in the first pilot stage of this initiative (Dix et al. 2012; Slee et al. 2009) concluded that:

- there were reduced mental health difficulties and increased mental health strengths in students, especially those who were rated as having higher levels of mental health difficulties at the start of the initiative;
- the average academic results of students in 'high implementing schools' were superior (by up to six months on National assessments on literacy and numeracy) to those of students in low implementation schools. This was over and above any influence of socioeconomic background. These results also supported anecdotal reports by participating teachers during the pilot that the school's implementation of their KidsMatter program had led to improvements in their students' schoolwork.

1.8 Positive Psychology and Positive Education

Positive psychology is a relatively new discipline in psychology. The goal of positive psychology is to provide the conditions and processes that contribute to optimal functioning in individuals, groups and institutions (Gable and Haidt 2005, p. 104). In positive psychology the emphasis is on individual and collective strengths rather than deficits, on positive experiences rather than problems, on competency building rather than pathology (Seligman and Csikszentmihalyi 2000). Positive psychology focuses on programs and interventions that contribute to wellbeing and happiness. One of the founders of positive psychology, Martin Seligman (2011) has developed the PERMA acronym to organise the five elements of wellbeing (Positive emotions, Engagement, Relationships, Meaning and Purpose and Accomplishment).

We offer a new acronym PROSPER as an organiser for the evidence-based positive psychological interventions that can help individuals, groups, organisations or communities to thrive. The term 'to prosper' is defined as to thrive and succeed in a healthy way; to flourish (*Oxford dictionary*; *Merriam-Webster Dictionary*). Thus the term 'PROSPER' encapsulates the goal of positive psychological interventions. The PROSPER acronym stands for Positivity, Relationships, Outcomes and accomplishment, Strengths, Purpose, Engagement, Resilience.

The PROSPER framework is similar to Seligman's PERMA model of wellbeing (Positive emotions, Engagement, Relationships, Meaning and Accomplishment) but includes two additional individual components: *Strengths* and *Resilience*. Resilience is considered an important indicator of wellbeing as illustrated in the model of flourishing adopted by Huppert and So (2013) as the basis of a tool for the measurement of the wellbeing of 43,000 citizens from twenty-three European countries. Their model of flourishing also includes components that are similar to those in the PROSPER model. The chart below highlights the similarities and differences between the PROSPER framework, the PERMA model and Huppert and So's model of flourishing (Table 1.1).

The component of Strengths is included in PROSPER because the deployment of one's strengths is seen as central to wellbeing theory (e.g. Seligman 2011) and because the awareness, development and application of students' character and ability strengths can be directly targeted within a school context.

The additional elements in the Huppert and So model: self-esteem, vitality and emotional stability have been subsumed in the PROSPER elements; emotional stability under Resilience and Vitality under Positivity. The construct self respect is included as a character strength in PROSPER replacing the construct of self esteem given the reported concerns with the self esteem construct. Seligman and his colleagues (Seligman et al. 1995) had highlighted some of the inadequacies of the concept of 'self-esteem' when they argued that:

> Armies of… teachers, along with… parents, are straining to bolster children's self esteem. That sounds innocuous enough, but the way they do it often erodes children's sense of worth. By emphasizing how a child feels, at the expense of what the child does-mastery,

Table 1.1   Comparing PROSPER framework with Hupper and So's (2013) model of flourishing and Seligman's (2011) PERMA model of flourishing

PROSPER framework	Hupper and So's model of flourishing	Seligman's PERMA model of flourishing
Positivity (positive emotions; positive mindset e.g. optimistic thinking)	Positive emotions Optimism	Positive emotions
Relationships (positive peer relationship and teacher-student relationships)	Relationships	Relationships
Outcomes	Competence	Accomplishment
Strengths (character strengths, ability strengths; self-respect)		
Purpose	Purpose	Meaning
Engagement	Engagement	Engagement
Resilience	Resilience	
	Self-esteem	
	Vitality	
	Emotional stability	

persistence, overcoming frustration and boredom and meeting a challenge-parents and teachers are making this generation of children more vulnerable to depression (p. 27)

As far back as 1996, Professor Roy Baumeister, formerly a strong advocate of the self esteem movement concluded that:

It is .....with considerable personal disappointment that I must report that the enthusiastic claims of the self-esteem movement mostly range from fantasy to hogwash. The effects of self-esteem are small, limited, and not all good.....And most of the time self-esteem makes surprisingly little difference (Baumeister et al. 1996, p. 14).

Baumeister and his colleagues (2005) later reported on the results of an analysis they conducted of all of the research studies on the impact of self-esteem that had been undertaken over the previous 35 years. They concluded that very little research to date has been able to demonstrate that enhancing self-esteem makes any difference to student learning and achievement or to the prevention of undesirable behavior in young people such as substance abuse, truancy, violence and promiscuity. However the concept of 'self-respect' (McGrath and Noble 2014) has been included under the component of 'Strengths'. Although self-respect and self-esteem are related concepts, they are also different. Self-esteem is an evaluation of one's 'worth' as a person and ranges from low to high self esteem. Self-esteem focuses more on successes, what one can do, what one looks like, and/or what one has. Therefore self-esteem fluctuates because it is usually very dependent on feedback from others. In contrast self-respect is an attitude of self-acceptance and approval for one's own character and conduct and consideration for one's own wellbeing.

Feedback on the theoretical and evidence-informed seven components of the PROSPER framework was provided by fifteen researchers and professors, at the Institute of Positive Psychology and Education (IPPE) at the Australian Catholic University. All IPPE members supported the inclusion of all seven components as well as providing constructive feedback on what they saw as the omission of some key elements (e.g. 'mindfulness' which has now been added to 'Positivity') from each of the seven components. Each component of PROSPER meets Seligman's three criteria for an element of wellbeing i.e. (i) each element contributes to wellbeing, (ii) each element can be defined and measured independently of the other elements and (iii) many people pursue the element for it's own sake (Seligman 2011 p. 16).

Feedback on the usefulness of the PROSPER framework was also sought from a convenience sample of educators. All of the teachers and principals who attended a one-day workshop on student wellbeing were asked for their feedback on the usefulness and relevance of the PROSPER framework at the end of the workshop. The compulsory workshop was inclusive of all teaching staff at four government primary schools, not just those teachers with designated responsibility for student wellbeing or social-emotional learning. The teachers were invited to respond anonymously to a seven-item questionnaire using a 5-point Likert scale from strongly disagree to strongly agree. Fifty-four respondents posted their survey responses face down in a box as they exited the workshop. Positive education was a new discipline for these schools and therefore the teachers were arguably less likely to have a preconceived idea of the usefulness or otherwise of a Positive Educational framework for their school practices. All respondents (100 %) agreed or strongly agreed that the PROSPER framework would help to provide a common language about wellbeing within their school and across schools. Most respondents (90 %) agreed or strongly agreed that it makes (a) the core components of wellbeing easy-to-remember and (b) is easy to communicate to everyone in their school community because of the relevant nature of the acronym. Most (96 %) also agreed or strongly agreed that the PROSPER framework would help staff to reflect on their practice for student wellbeing and 89 % also agreed or strongly agreed that the framework has the potential as an audit tool for identifying their school's current successful practices for student wellbeing as well as identifying the gaps. An assessment tool for measuring the PROSPER components for student wellbeing is under development.

In the next section we apply the PROSPER framework to the educational context. This application of PROSPER in education seems timely given Seligman's recent challenge to policy makers to develop a new measure of prosperity, beginning early in life. Seligman (2011) states:

> the time has come for a new prosperity, one that takes flourishing seriously as a the goal for education and of parenting. Learning to value and to attain flourishing must start early - in the formative years of schooling - and it is this new prosperity, kindled by positive education, that the world can now choose (Seligman 2011 p. 97).

In this publication the PROSPER framework will be applied to organising the evidence-based school practices that have the potential to enhance student well-being and achievement and build schools as enabling institutions. The PROSPER organiser builds on the authors' two earlier versions of a positive psychology framework for education. The first prototype evolved as an outcome of the authors' co-development of the Australian Government Scoping Study on Approaches to

Student Wellbeing (Noble and McGrath 2008) and the second prototype is titled the Positive Educational Practices (PEPs) Framework (Noble et al. 2008). PROSPER has some similarities with Geelong Grammar School's (GGS) Positive Education framework outlined by Norrish (2015). The GGS' domains are Positive Emotions, Positive Relationships, Positive Accomplishment, Character Strengths, Positive Purpose, Positive Engagement and Positive Health and Resilience.

1.8.1 Our Definition of Positive Education

Here positive education is defined as:

> the integration of the core principles of Positive Psychology with the evidence-informed structures, practices and programs that enhance both wellbeing and academic achievement. The aim of positive education is to enable all members of a school community to succeed and prosper

1.9 The PROSPER Framework for Student Wellbeing

The PROSPER Student Wellbeing Framework represents the integration of the main ideas in Positive Psychology with the most up-to-date scientific knowledge about student wellbeing and social and emotional learning. It is a flexible framework, not a program. It has been designed as a guide for professional staff in early learning centres, primary schools and secondary schools who wish to implement a Positive Education approach at any or all of these levels.

Figure 1.1 outlines the PROSPER acronym and illustrates each of the seven components that contribute to wellbeing.

PROSPER:

Positivity. Positive mindset *(e.g. gratitude; optimistic thinking;positive tracking mindfulness) and* Positive emotions *(e.g. fun & enjoyment, satisfaction, safety, pride)*

Relationships *(e.g. prosocial values and social skills for developing positive relationships)*

Outcomes *(e.g. achievement; mastery; grit; goal setting; growth mindset etc)*

Strengths *(e.g. self-knowledge; self respect; awareness of one's character strengths; ability strengths; collective strengths)*

Purpose *(Having a sense of purpose through the pursuit of worthwhile goals both for the wellbeing of oneself and the wellbeing of others)*

Engagement *('psychological flow'; social, emotional, behavioural & cognitive)*

Resilience *(e.g. coping skills; self-management skills; courage)*

Fig. 1.1 The PROSPER framework

Chapter 2 employs the PROSPER organiser to outline the evidence-based school pathways that contribute to student wellbeing and to developing schools as supportive and safe school communities.

References

Adelman, H. S., & Taylor, L. (2003). On sustainability of project innovations as systemic change. *Journal of Educational and Psychological Consultation, 14*(1), 1–25.

Albright, M. I., & Weissberg, R. P. (2010). Family-school partnerships to promote social and emotional learning. In S. L. Christenson & A. L. Reschly (Eds.), *Handbook of school-family partnerships* (pp. 246–265). New York, NY: Routledge.

Albright, M. I., Weissberg, R. P., & Dusenbury, L. A. (2011). *School-family partnership strategies to enhance children's social, emotional, and academic growth.* Newton, MA: National Center for Mental Health Promotion and Youth Violence Prevention, Education Development Center, Inc.

Axford, S., Schepens, R., & Blyth, K. (2011). Did introducing the bounce back programme have an impact on resilience, connectedness and wellbeing of children and teachers in 16 primary schools in Perth and Kinross, Scotland? *Educational Psychology, 12*(1), 2–5.

Bandura, A. (1996). Exercise of personal and collective efficacy in changing societies. In A. Bandura (Ed.), *Self-efficacy in changing societies* (pp. 1–45). NY: Cambridge Press.

Barrett, P. M., Cooper, M., & Teoh, B. H. (2014). When time is of the essence: A rationale for 'earlier' early intervention. *Journal of Psychological Abnormalities in Children, 3*(4), 1–9.

Barry, M.A., Clarke, A.M., Jenkins, R., & Patel, V. (2013). A systematic review of the effectiveness of mental health promotion interventions for young people in low and middle income countries. *BMC Public Health, 13*, 835. http://www.biomedcentral.com/1471-2458/13/835.

Baumeister, R. F., Campbell, J. D., Krueger, J. I., & Vohs, K. D. (2005). Exploding the self-esteem Myth. *Scientific American Mind, 16*(4), 50–57.

Baumeister, R. F., Smart, L., & Boden, J. (1996). The dark side of high self-esteem. *Psychological Review, 68*, 70–71.

Browne, G., Gafni, A., Roberts, J., Byrne, C., & Mujumbar, B. (2004). Effective/efficient mental health programs for school-age children: A synthesis of reviews. *Social Science and Medicine, 58*, 1367–1384.

Catalano, R. F., Mazzab, J. J., Harachia, T. W., Abbott, R. D., Haggerty, K. P., & Fleminga, C. B. (2003). Raising healthy children through enhancing social development in elementary school: Results after 1.5 years. *Journal of School Psychology, 41*(2), 143–164.

Catalano, R. F., Kosterman, R., Hawkins, J. D., et al. (1996). Modelling the etiology of adolescent substance use: A test of the social development model. *Journal of Drug Issues, 26*, 429–455.

Datnow, A., & Castellano, M. (2000). Teachers' responses to success for all: How beliefs, experiences, and adaptations shape implementation. *American Educational Research Journal, 37*, 775.

De Fraine, B., Van Landeghem, G., & Van Damme, J. (2005). An analysis of well-being in secondary school with multilevel growth curve models and multilevel multivariate models. *Quality & Quantity, 39*, 297–316.

Delors, J. (1996). Learning the treasure within. Report to UNESCO of the International Commission on Education for the Twenty-first Century.

Diekstra, R. F. W., & Gravesteijn, C. (2008). Effectiveness of school-based social and emotional education programmes worldwide. http://www.lions-quest.org/pdfs/EvaluationBotinEnglish.pdf.

Dix, K. L., Slee, P. T., Lawson, M. J. & Keeves, J. P. (2012). Implementation quality of whole school mental health promotion and students' academic performance. *Child Adolescence Mental Health, 17*(1), 45–51.

Durlak, J. A. (2015). What everyone should know about implementation. In J. A. Durlak., C. E. Domitrovich., R. P. Weissberg., T. P. Gullotta (Eds.), *Handbook of Social and Emotional Learning*. New York: The Guildford Press.

Durlak, J. A., Weissberg, R. P., Dymnicki, A. B., Taylor, R. D., & Schellinger, K. B. (2011). The impact of enhancing students' social and emotional learning: A meta-analysis of school-based universal interventions. *Child Development, 82*(1), 405–432.

Eckert, T. L., & Hintz, J. M. (2000). Behavioral conceptions and applications of acceptability: Issues related to service delivery and research methodology. *School Psychology Quarterly, 15*, 123–148.

Elias, M. (2003). Academic and social-emotional learning. *International Academy of Education, 1, 5–3*, 1.

Elias, J. E., Zins, P. A., Graczyk, R. P., & Weissberg, R. (2003). Implementation, sustainability, and scaling up of social-emotional and academic innovations in public schools. *School Psychology Review, 32*, 303.

Engels, N., Aelterman, A., Van Petegem, K., & Schepens, A. (2004). Factors which influence the well-being of pupils in Flemish secondary schools. *Educational Studies, 30*(2), 127–143. Engelwood Cliffs, NJ: Prentice-Hall.

Fraillon, J. (2004). *Measuring Student Wellbeing in the Context of Australian Schooling: Discussion Paper* Commissioned by the South Australian Department of Education and Children's services as an agent of the Ministerial Council on Education, Employment, Training and Youth Affairs. http://www.mceetya.edu.au/verve/_resources/Measuring_Student_Well-Being_in_the_Context_of_Australian_Schooling.pdf.

Gable, S. J., & Haidt, J. (2005). What (and why) is positive psychology? *Review of General Psychology, 9*(2), 103–110.

Gillham, J., Brunwasser, S. M., & Freres, D. R. (2008). Preventing depression in early adolescence: The penn resiliency program. In J. R. Z. Abela & B. L. Hankin (Eds.), *Handbook of depression in children and adolescents* (pp. 309–332). New York: Guilford.

Global Burden of Disease Study 2010. (2012). *Global burden of diseases, injuries, and risk factors study 2010*. Seattle: Institute for Health, Metrics and Evaluation.

Gottfredson, L. S. (1998). The general intelligence factor. *Scientific American Presents, 9*(4), 24–29.

Greenberg, M. T., Domitrovich, C., & Bumbarger, B. (2001). *Preventing mental disorders in school-age children: A review of the effectiveness of prevention programs*. Report commissioned by the Center for Mental Health Services (CMHS), Substance Abuse Mental Health Services Administration, US Department of Health and Human Services.

Greenberg, M., Weissberg, R., O'Brien, M., Zins, J., Fredericks, L., Resnik, H., & Elias, M. (2003). Enhancing school-based prevention and youth development through coordinated social, emotional, and academic learning. *American Psychologist, 58*, 466–474.

Gresham, F. M., & Lopez, M. F. (1996). Social validation: A unifying concept for school-based consultation research and practice. *School Psychology Quarterly, 11*(3), 204–227.

Griffin, P., McGaw, B., & Care, E. (Eds.). (2012). *Assessment and teaching of 21st century skills*. Springer: Dordrecht.

Han, S. S., & Weiss, B. (2005). Sustainability of teacher implementation of school-based mental health programs. *Journal of Abnormal Child Psychology, 33*(6), 665–679.

Hassall, I., & Hanna, K. (2007). *School-based violence prevention programme*. A literature review: Accident compensation corporation.

Hattie, J. (2009). *Visible learning: A synthesis of over 800 meta-analyses relating to achievement*. London: Routledge.

Huppert, F. A., & So, T. T. C. (2013) Flourishing across europe: Application of a new conceptual framework for defining well-being. *Social Indicators Research, 110*(3), 837–861.

Johnson, D. W., Johnson, R. T., & Stanne, M. B. (2001). Cooperative learning methods: A meta-analysis. http://www.co-operation.org/pages/cl-methods.html.

Kam, C. M., Greenberg, M. T., & Walls, C. T. (2003). Examining the role of implementation quality in school-based prevention using the PATHS curriculum. *Prevention Science, 4*, 55–63.

Kim, E. M., Coutts, M. J., Holmes, S. R., Sheridan, S. M., Ransom, K. A., Sjuts, T. M., & Rispoli, K. M. (2012). *Parent involvement and family-school partnerships: Examining the content, processes, and outcomes of structural versus relationship-based approaches.* CYS Working Paper 2012-6, Nebraska Center for Research: Children, Youth families & Schools. Downloaded 11 February 2015 from: http://files.eric.ed.gov/fulltext/ED537851.pdf.

Kim-Cohen, J., Caspi, A., Moffitt, T. E., Harrington, H., Milne, B. J., & Poulton, R. (2003). Prior juvenile diagnoses in adults with mental disorder: Developmental follow-back of a prospective-longitudinal cohort. *Archives of General Psychiatry, 60*, 709–717.

Layard, R., & Hagell, A. (2015). Healthy young minds: Transforming the mental health of children. In J. H. Helliwell, R. Layard & J.Sachs (Eds.), *World Happiness Report 2015.* New York: Sustainable Development Solutions Network. www.unsdsn.org/happiness.

Luby, J. L. (2010). Preschool depression: The importance of identification of depression early in development. *Current Directions in Psychological Science, 19*, 91–95.

McGrath, H., & Francey, S. (1991). *Friendly kids, friendly classrooms.* Melbourne: Pearson Education. (Nastasi, 2002).

McGrath, H., & Noble, T. (2003). *BOUNCE back! A classroom resiliency program. Teacher's handbook.* Sydney: Pearson Education.

McGrath, H., & Noble, T. (2011). *BOUNCE BACK! A wellbeing & resilience program. Lower primary K-2; middle primary: Yrs 3-4; upper primary/junior secondary: Yrs 5-8.* Melbourne: Pearson Education.

Marzano, R. J., Pickering, D. J., & Pollock, J. E. (2001). *Classroom instruction that works: Research-based strategies for increasing student achievement.* Alexandria, VA: Association for Supervision and Curriculum Development.

New Development Paradigm. (2013). *NDP steering committee and secretariat. Happiness: Towards a new development paradigm.* Report of the Kingdom of Bhutan. Royal Government of Bhutan. http://www.newdevelopmentparadigm.bt/.

Noble, T., & McGrath, H. (2008). The positive educational practices framework : A tool for facilitating the work of educational psychologists in promoting pupil wellbeing. *Educational and child psychology, 25*(2), 119–134.

Noble, T., McGrath, H. L. Roffey, S. & Rowling, L. (2008). *Scoping study into approaches to student wellbeing: A report to the department of education, employment and workplace relations.*

Noble, T. & McGrath, H. (2014). Wellbeing and resilience in school settings. In C. Ruini & G. A. Fava (Eds.), *Increasing psychological wellbeing across cultures.* New York, NY: Springer.

Norrish, J. (2015). *Positive education. The Geelong Grammar School Journey.* Oxford: Oxford University Press.

NSSF: National Safe Schools Framework. (2011). http://www.deewr.gov.au/schooling/nationalsafeschools/Pages/overview.aspx.

OECD. (2014). *Making mental health count: The social and economic costs of neglecting mental health care, OECD health policy studies.* Paris: OECD Publishing.

O'Malley, M., Katz, K., Renshaw, T., & Furlong, M. (2012). Gauging the system: Trends in school climate measurement and intervention. In S. Jimerson, A. Nickerson, M. Mayer, & M. Furlong (Eds.), *The handbook of school violence and school safety: International research and practice* (2nd ed., pp. 317–329). New York: Routledge.

O'Shaughnessy, T. E., Lane, K. E., Gresham, F. E., & Beebe-Frankenberge, M. E. (2003). Children placed at risk for learning and behavioral difficulties. Implementing a school-wide system of early identification and intervention. *Remedial and Special Education, 24*(1), 27–35.

Reivich, K. (2005). Lecture on resilience. *Authentic Happiness Coaching Online Course.*

Resnick, M. D., Bearman, P. S., & Blum, R. W. (1997). Protecting adolescents from harm: Findings from the national longitudinal study on adolescent health. *JAMA, 278*, 823–832.

Roseth, C. J., Johnson, D. W., & Johnson, R. T. (2008). Promoting early adolescents' achievement and peer relationships: The effects of cooperative, competitive and individualistic goal structures. *Psychological Bulletin, 134*(2), 223–246.

Ryan, R. M., & Deci, E. L. (2001). On happiness and human potentials: A review of research on hedonic and eudaimonic well-being. In S. Fiske (Ed.), *Annual review of psychology* (Vol. 52, pp. 141–166). Palo Alto, CA: Annual Reviews Inc.

Seligman, M. E. P. (1998). *Learned optimism*. New York: Knopf.

Seligman, M. E. (2011). *Flourish: A visionary new understanding of happiness and wellbeing*. NY: Simon and Schuster.

Seligman, M. P., & Csikszentmihalyi, M. (2000). Positive psychology. *American Psychologist, 55*, 5–14.

Seligman, M. E. P., Reivich, K., Jaycox, L., & Gillham, J. (1995). *The optimistic child*. New York: Houghton Mifflin.

Shonkoff, J., & Phillips, D. (Eds.). (2000). *From neurons to neighborhoods: The science of early childhood development*. Washington, DC: National Academy Press.

Slee, P. T., Lawson, M .J., Russell, A., Askell-Williams, H., Dix, K. L., Owens, L. D., Skrzypiec, G., & Spears. (2009). KidsMatter primary evaluation final report B. http://dspace2.flinders.edu.au/xmlui/handle/2328/26832

Sugai, G., Horner, R., & Lewis, T. (2009). *School-wide positive behaviour support implementers' blueprint and self-assessment*. Eugene, OR: OSEP TA-Center on Positive Behavioral Interventions and Supports.

UNICEF. (2014). *The state of the world's children 2014 in numbers*. Available from www.unicef.org/sowc2014/numbers/.

Webster-Stratton, C., & Taylor, T. (2001). Nipping early risk factors in the bud: Preventing substance abuse, delinquency, and violence in adolescence through interventions targeted at young children (ages 0–8 years). *Prevention Science, 2*(3), 165–192.

Weissberg, R. P., & O'Brien, M. U. (2004). What works in school-based social and emotional learning programs for positive youth development. *Annals of the American Academy of Political and Social Science, 591*, 86–97.

Wells, J., Barlow, J., & Stewart-Brown, S. (2003). A systematic review of universal approaches to mental health promotion in schools. *Health Education, 103*(4), 197–220.

World Health Organisation (WHO). (2003). *Caring for children and adolescent with mental disorders: Setting WHO directions*. Geneva: World Health Organisation.

Zins, J. E., Weissberg, R. P., Wang, M. C., & Walberg, H. J. (Eds.). (2004). *Building academic success on social and emotional learning: What does the research say?*. New York: Teachers College Press.

Chapter 2
The Prosper Framework for Student Wellbeing

Abstract This chapter introduces the PROSPER school pathways for student wellbeing. Sustainable student wellbeing is seen as an outcome of the school policies, structures and practices that are organized under the PROSPER framework. The research evidence for each PROSPER school pathway is discussed: Encouraging **P**ositivity, Building **R**elationships, Facilitating **O**utcomes, Focusing on **S**trengths, Fostering a sense of **P**urpose and Teaching **R**esilience. Case studies and Boxes that illustrate the research into practice are also included. Chapter two concludes with a series of questions that encourages school practitioners to reflect on their capacity to implement Positive Education structures, processes and practices in their schools. Using the term PROSPER easily communicates the purpose of a school framework for student wellbeing.

Keywords Positive education · Positivity · Relationships · Outcomes · Strengths · Purpose · Engagement resilience

PROSPER is employed in this section as an organizer for the school factors that contribute to student wellbeing and their engagement in learning. All the PROSPER wellbeing components and the school practices outlined in the following section are derived from the positive psychological literature as well as the educational psychological literature. PROSPER in the school context is not a program but an organizing framework for the evidence-based school and classroom practices that facilitate student wellbeing and build safe and supportive school communities. The more PROSPER components that a student is able to access at school, the better their education and the higher their level of wellbeing and achievement is likely to be. Sustainable student wellbeing is seen as an outcome of the school policies, structures and practices that are organized under the PROSPER framework.

© The Author(s) 2016   25
T. Noble and H. McGrath, *The PROSPER School Pathways for Student Wellbeing,*
SpringerBriefs in Well-Being and Quality of Life Research,
DOI 10.1007/978-3-319-21795-6_2

2.1   Introducing the PROSPER Framework in the School Context

Positivity for students means experiencing positive emotions at school such as feeling safe, a sense of belonging, interested, content and cheerful and experiencing a sense of fun and amusement. Positivity also incorporates a gratitude and appreciation, positive mindset that includes a capacity for mindfulness and skills in optimistic thinking.

Relationships for students means experiencing ongoing positive relationships with peers and teachers; for parents it means experiencing ongoing positive relationship with teachers and the school; for teachers it means experiencing ongoing positive relationships with other school staff parents and their students. A focus on building positive relationships also means teaching the prosocial values and the social skills that enable such relationships and on identifying and implementing school-based structures that facilitate these relationships.

Outcomes involves making progress toward goals, feeling capable to do schoolwork, understanding that accomplishment depends on hard work and effort, being persistent, and having a 'growth mindset', and a sense of mastery and achievement. There is a focus on teaching these attitudes and skills, using evidence-informed teaching strategies that facilitate both positive school-based outcomes (both academic and co-curricular). There is also a focus on acknowledging and celebrating the accomplishment of all members of the school community in a wide range of school-based outcomes.

Strengths involves self knowledge about one's character strengths and ability strengths and understanding how to apply these strengths in different contexts; there is a focus on assisting all members of the school community to identify their strengths, develop them further and find good ways to apply their strengths.

Purpose in the school context refers to believing that what one is learning at school is valuable and feeling connected to something greater than oneself; there is also a focus on looking for ways to be of service to the school community, to the general community and to people in need of care and support.

Engagement refers to student's psychological connection to learning activities and to school (e.g. feeling absorbed, connected, interested, and engaged in school learning and in school life); there is also a focus on effective and evidence-informed teaching strategies for enhancing student engagement.

Resilience includes having the capacity to 'bounce back' after setbacks, mistakes and difficulties and being courageous when faced with challenging situations; there is also a focus on explicitly teaching coping skills and implementing support structures.

Section 2.2 provides an overview of the evidence base for each of the PROSPER school components and then offers some practical classroom or school examples of how each component can be implemented in classrooms and schools. The following table provides a summary of how each PROSPER component provides an organizer for the strategies that each school can implement to foster student wellbeing (Table 2.1).

Table 2.1 The PROSPER School Pathways

PROSPER school pathways	Examples of school and classroom practices and structures
Encouraging POSITIVITY Supporting students to develop a positive mindset and experience positive emotions	• Provision of opportunities for students to experience and amplify positive emotions and build positive learning environments e.g. through the use of music, dance, humour, cooperative learning tasks • Explicit teaching of the values and skills needed for a Positive Mindset – Optimistic thinking, positive tracking, positive conversion, hopeful thinking and expressing gratitude – Mindfulness • Provision of opportunities to practise these skills
Building RELATIONSHIPS Supporting students to develop the social skills and pro-social values that underpin positive relationships and building positive relationships within the school	• Strategies for developing: – A safe and supportive school culture – Positive student–teacher relationships – Positive student-peer relationships – Positive school-family and school-community relationships • Explicit teaching of social skills and pro-social values • Provision of opportunities to practise these skills • Interpersonal structures that facilitate relationships e.g. cooperative learning groups, circle time cross-age teams, cooperative games and performance groups
Facilitating OUTCOMES Provision of optimal learning environments and opportunities to learn specific skills that enhance students' outcomes and accomplishment	• Adoption of evidence-informed teaching strategies • Explicit teaching of skills for: – Organisation – Goal achievement (e.g. *effort, persistence + willpower (grit) and problem-solving*) – Effective studying • Promotion of a growth mindset • The use of critical and creative thinking tools
Focusing on STRENGTHS Taking a strengths-based approach with students, teachers and the whole school community	Adoption of strengths-based approaches to organisation, curriculum and planning which results in: • Student self knowledge in relation to strengths • Opportunities for students to further develop and use/demonstrate their strengths • Task differentiation based on students' character and ability strengths • Recognition and application of teacher and parent strengths and collective strengths
Fostering a sense of PURPOSE Supporting students to develop a sense of purpose and meaning	Provision of opportunities for students to: • Participate in student-owned and student-directed activities • Be involved with community service or service learning • Make contributions to the school through 'student voice' and participation in decision-making about aspects of the school • Undertake roles requiring peer mentoring or peer support • Undertake leadership roles • Explore spirituality
Enhancing ENGAGEMENT Providing opportunities for high student engagement	Adoption of: • Evidence-informed teaching and learning strategies • Relationship-based teaching strategies • Activities that incorporate critical and creative thinking • Curriculum differentiation so students experience 'flow'
Teaching RESILIENCE Supporting students to develop the skills and attitudes that underpin resilient behaviour	Explicit teaching of skills for: • Coping and acting resiliently in both personal and academic contexts • Acting with courage • Good decision-making • Self management

2.2   PROSPER Pathway 1: Encouraging POSITIVITY

Positivity can be defined simply *'as the state or character of being positive; a positivity that accepts the world as it is'* (Dictionary.com; 2014). The term 'positivity' is employed by Fredrickson (2009, p. 6) to include the positive meanings and optimistic attitudes that trigger positive emotions. Positivity also incorporates the long-term impact that positive emotions have on one's character, relationships, communities and environment. According to the British Cohort Study the best predictor of a child becoming a satisfied and happy adult is not their academic achievement but their emotional health in childhood (Layard and Hagell 2015). A focus on Positivity (see Table 2.1) encourages educators to provide the classroom and school opportunities to develop student's emotional health. For example enabling students to experience and amplify positive emotions such as feeling connected, feeling safe and feeling amused. Amplifying emotions means 'turning them up' to maximise their effect and consciously 'savouring' them. Helping students to develop a 'Positivity mindset' also requires educators to explicitly teach students the values and skills associated with positivity such as expressing gratitude and thinking optimistically.

2.2.1   Positive Emotions

What role do positive emotions play in helping students, groups or schools to thrive? A great deal of research under the positive psychology umbrella has shown that people who experience and express positive emotions more frequently than others are more resilient (Fredrickson and Tugade 2004), resourceful (Lyubomirsky et al. 2005), socially connected (Mauss et al. 2011), and more likely to function at optimal levels (Fredrickson and Losada 2005; Mauss et al. 2011). Fredrickson's (2013) 'broaden and build' model is helpful in understanding the key role of positive emotions for optimal functioning and prospering. The model proposes that even brief experiences of positive emotions such as interest, joy, security, gratitude, hopefulness and amusement can both broaden an individual's thoughts and actions and accumulate over time in ways that can incrementally contribute to an individual's collection of personal resources that can be employed as needed to enhance their resilience, confidence and relationships.

Understanding the significant role that positive emotions can play in schools and the impact they can have on learning and wellbeing is the starting point for schools to design policies, programs, structures and strategies that can ensure that students experience a range of positive emotions on a regular basis. We discuss the role of feelings of belonging, feeling safe, feeling satisfied in learning and feeling amused.

(i) *Feelings of belonging and connectedness.* Belonging is one of the most significant factors that schools can build to improve the lives of their students across a host of outcomes. In a large study of over 12,000 adolescents school connectedness emerged as one of the two most consistent and powerful protective factors against every measured form of adolescent risk and distress (Resnick et al. 1997). The other factor was family connectedness. The need to belong and feel connected (defined as 'relatedness' by Ryan and Deci 2000) is seen as one of the three basic human needs according to self determination theory. The other two needs identified in self determination theory are competence and autonomy. Goodenow (1993) described a student's sense of belonging at school as not only being liked and treated with warmth but also a:

> ... sense of being accepted, valued, included, and encouraged by others (teacher and peers) in the academic classroom setting and of feeling oneself to be an important part of the life and activity of the class. .....it also involves support and respect for personal autonomy and for the student as an individual. (p. 25)

A review of research (Becker and Luthar 2002) concluded that a sense of belonging at school is a key factor that contributes to the classroom engagement and academic motivation of middle school students from economically disadvantaged and/or minority backgrounds. For example, the students' sense of belonging to their school emerged as the central and significant variable in explaining student psychological wellbeing in a study of almost 700 students in two high schools. In this study the more connected the students felt, the less likely they were to report feelings of anxiety, depression and display angry aggression and the less likely their teachers were to rate their behaviour as disruptive (Bizumic et al. 2009).

A review of the research by Osterman (2000) and studies by Blum and Libbey (2004a, b), and Militich et al. (2004) suggest that students who have a sense of belonging and connectedness at school are more likely to:

- actively participate at school, be more interested and engaged with classroom and school activities, show more commitment to their school and their schoolwork and have a positive orientation towards school and teachers
- act supportively towards peers and demonstrate more pro-social behaviour
- have higher expectations for their own success
- demonstrate greater acceptance of authority
- accept more responsibility for regulating their own behaviour in the classroom
- achieve more highly through the indirect effects of higher levels of participation, interest and engagement and be less likely to drop our early from school

Furrer and Skinner (2003) found that students who had a strong sense of belonging also demonstrated higher levels of academic motivation, enthusiasm and both behavioural and emotional engagement with school. In contrast, those students who felt unimportant or ignored by teachers reported more unhappiness, boredom and anger when participating in classroom learning activities. Furrer and Skinner suggested that a sense of relatedness may function as a motivational resource for students when they are confronted by a challenge or difficulty. Other studies (e.g. Newman 1991) have identified positive associations between adolescents' sense of belonging at school and academic help-seeking behaviour. Joyce and Early (2014) surveyed 1852 adolescents across 132 schools and identified that higher school connectedness and getting along with teachers were significantly associated with having fewer symptoms of depression.

Student-focused classroom environments (*characterised by student cohesiveness and support for each other, friendly teacher support, student involvement with decision-making about learning tasks, the use of investigation, peer cooperation, the extent to which the teacher treats students equally*) was positively associated with student avoidance of self-handicapping behaviours such as putting off a homework task or study until the last moment and deliberately not trying to do well on learning tasks (Dorman and Ferguson 2004). Students who feel a strong sense of connection to their school are also less likely to engage in health-compromising behaviour (e.g. Bond et al. 2001). On the other hand, when students experience negative feelings such as grief, jealousy, anger and loneliness associated with a lack of belonging, rejection or isolation, they are less likely to conform to school rules and norms (Wentzel and Asher 1995) and more likely to have negative perceptions of school and schoolwork, avoid school and leave school at an early age (Ladd 1990).

Classroom and school-based approaches that have the potential to increase a students' sense of belonging include:

- Maximising opportunities for students to work together in small groups so that they can share ideas and get to know each other (Jones and Gerig 1994).
- Using co-operative learning approaches for instruction. Osterman (2000) has argued that cooperative learning is especially effective as it increases the frequency of positive student interactions each day.
- Looking for opportunities to let students know that they are cared for. Baumeister and Leary (1995) have argued that a student's perception that they are cared about and supported is especially significant in creating a sense of belonging. This feeling can be developed in a range of ways such as: celebrating birthdays, sending home 'get well' cards when students are absent and establishing peer support structures such as cross age buddies, peer tutoring and peer mediators (Stanley and McGrath 2006).

Bower et al. (2014) investigated approaches to developing student social connectedness in three Australian high schools. All three schools used school-wide practices to involve the school community in the education process, taking into account the importance of cultural and background differences. Areas that were identified by teachers as being important for further improving students' social connectedness included using technology for building community and ensuring that teachers had opportunities for professional learning that would enable them to explicitly teach key social and emotional skills to their students.

(ii) *Feelings of safety.* Students are most likely to report feeling safe in schools that have low levels of putdowns and bullying and in which students feel confident that if they ask a teacher for assistance with dealing with a bullying session then they will be supported and the bullying will be stopped. All students feel less safe when they know that unchecked bullying is occurring in their school, even if they haven't been targets for this kind of behaviour themselves (e.g. Janson et al. 2009). Felson et al. (1994) found that tacit approval for the use of aggression in a school (e.g. through bullying) was associated with students' placing less value on academic achievement. Overall levels of achievement in both reading and maths have been found to be lower in schools with higher levels of bullying (Konishi et al. 2010). Feeling safe at school from being bullied or taunted allows students to give their full attention to their relationships and schoolwork rather than always being alert to potential threats to their wellbeing.

Bullying occurs at some level in all primary and secondary schools (Elias and Zins 2003) and all students can potentially become involved in bullying others or being bullied. Many students report occasionally taking part in some form of bullying and most students are teased or experience some form of peer harassment during their years at school (e.g. Espelage and Swearer 2003) However bullying can cause great suffering and can adversely affect a students' mental health and academic outcomes. It can also cause harm to the students who engage in bullying behaviour. Students who bully others frequently, as well as students who are bullied, are more likely to feel disconnected from school and to dislike school (Cross et al. 2009).

The explicit teaching and development of the social-emotional skills related to empathy should be part of this picture. Observing the distress of others and responding to it with empathy is what inhibits most students from taking part in bullying (Endresen and Olweus (2001). Those students who often take part in bullying have been found to be more likely to have lower levels of empathy than other students (Espelage et al. 2004; Gini et al. 2007; Jolliffe and Farrington 2006). A further argument for the implementation of a preventative approach that includes the teaching of pro-social values, social and emotional skills and resilience skills has emerged from studies such as that of Bosworth et al. (1999). They found that children who are the angriest within a classroom are also the most likely to bully others. Similarly Swearer and Cary (2007) found that students who often bullied others reported that the primary reason for their bullying behaviour was their need to relieve stress or not coping well when 'having a bad day'.

A meta-analysis of 30 well-designed evaluations of anti-bullying interventions identifies the specific components that appear to have had the greatest impact on decreasing bullying behaviour (Farrington and Ttofi 2009). The researchers concluded that the most effective anti-bullying programs reduced bullying incidents by an average of 20–23 %. The specific components that made the most impact were:

- Clear classroom and school rules against bullying that are consistently enforced and re-stated
- Intensive professional learning for teachers
- Effective classroom management
- Improved playground/yard supervision
- School conferences or assemblies that raised awareness of the problem
- The use of effective behaviour management strategies and the provision of training for teachers in their implementation

- Student-owned and student-directed approaches to prevent bullying.
- The use of video educational material for students
- Parent education about bullying

They also found that the most effective interventions were multi-faceted, of longer duration and involved school collaboration with other appropriate professionals in working with individual students.

Bullying is a multifaceted problem that requires a multifaceted solution (see NSSF 2011a, b). The first aspect to focus on in the prevention of bullying is through specific rules about 'no bullying' coupled with a preventative anti-bullying curriculum. The second aspect to focus on is equipping all school staff (including visiting and temporary replacement teachers) with the knowledge and skills that they need in order to manage any bullying situations in a fair but firm manner and to support those students who have been mistreated. The third aspect to focus on is the implementation of the components of the PROSPER framework that contribute to a positive and supportive school climate. Low levels of bullying are more likely in schools in which there is effective school leadership which articulates a vision for whole school wellbeing underpinned by pro-social values (such as respect and acceptance of differences) and an effective and consistent whole school positive behaviour management program (McGrath 2007).

(iii) *Feelings of satisfaction, affirmation and pride in learning & school life.* Students experience feelings of pride and satisfaction when they have opportunities to experience success and when their school focuses on the celebration of those successes. To provide such opportunities schools need to value different kinds of achievements (such as peer support or volunteering) and not just success in the traditional academic or sports domains (Kornhaber et al. 2003; Noble 2004). See Outcomes for more discussion on students experiencing success at school.

(iv) *Feeling amused and experiencing fun and enjoyment.* The provision of a range of activities that offer students opportunities to experience the positive emotions of amusement, and enjoyment through having fun has many benefits in terms of student wellbeing and classroom wellbeing. Laughter relaxes and calms the body and enhances pleasure and positive mood through the release of dopamine into the brain (Martin 2006). Laughter also has the capacity to reduce stress (Bennett and Lengacher 2008; Colom et al. 2011) and improve the functioning of the immune system (Berk 2001). Finding the humorous side or participating in humour-based activities can sometimes be an effective strategy for coping resiliently with difficult times in one's life and for reducing anxiety (Booth-Butterfield et al. 2007; Yovetich et al. 1990). A review of several studies into the positive effects of humour in educational contexts concluded that the use of non-aggressive positive humour can contribute to a more engaging and relaxed learning environment, enhance student's positive perceptions of the teacher who employs it, increase students' motivation to learn about the content of the lesson, and result in more overall enjoyment of the lesson content and tasks (Banas et al. 2011). Some research studies have found that humour can also enhance the learning and recall of information and creative thinking (e.g. see Morrison 2008). Teachers who make learning 'fun' are also more often liked and respected especially by boys (e.g. Keddie and Churchill 2003). Neuliep (1991) has proposed that, when used appropriately, humour can help to reduce some of the status-distance between teachers and students in a positive and warm way.

Humour can be used in many ways within a classroom context. It can be an interpersonal style adopted by a teacher when interacting with students or the class as a whole. It can be an approach to teaching and learning such as using humorous cartoons or images in a slide presentation or showing a short funny video clip that has some relevance to a topic. Humour can be built into a curriculum activity such as practising the relevant mathematics skills by conducting, collating and analysing the results of a class (or schoolwide) survey to identify the funniest of four different jokes or six funny stories written by class groups. When used appropriately humour can also be used as an effective coping skill. For example a teacher might make a joke of it when he or a student makes a silly mistake to help keep things in perspective.

2.2.2   Positive Mindset

A positive mindset incorporates the following attitudes and skills:

(i) *Positive tracking*: This skill involves looking for and commenting on the positives that you encounter in your own life (however small) and in the actions of other people.

(ii) *Positive conversion*: This skill involves finding small positive aspects, opportunities and learning experiences in negative events and mistakes that occur in your life

(iii) *Using an optimistic explanatory style* (Seligman 1991, 1995): This is the skill of explaining and interpreting setbacks and difficult times in your life in a way that makes it more likely that you can cope well with them and move on from them. This involves:

   • Seeing bad times as temporary ('*just now*') rather than permanent ('*always*')
   • Perceiving that most setbacks and difficult times are 'temporary' ('*things will get better*'), they happen to other people too ('*not just me*') and are limited to the immediate incident not the whole of your life ('*just this*').

(iv) *Having a Sense of Hope*: Hopefulness has been shown to contribute to success and wellbeing (Lopez et al. 2009; Snyder and Lopez 2007). It contributes energy to goal-seeking and achievement. Hopefulness is important to the achievement of all types of goals such as learning goals, social goals, physical goals and performance goals.

People who feel hopeful about achieving what they want have a positive orientation that incorporates three key components, all of which can be explicitly taught to students. Hopeful people:

- have clear, specific and achievable goals that they are really motivated to achieve; they are also able to articulate why they want to achieve these goals
- look for flexible strategies/pathways to help them to achieve their goals and respond constructively to obstacles that might get in the way
- sustain their motivation and confidence to achieve their goals by using positive self-talk about their ability and capacity for hard work and they remind themselves about why they want to achieve this goal

Finding hope in difficult times: This skill focuses on believing that when an outcome of a worrying or stressful situation is unclear, it is still possible that things will turn out okay

(v) *Gratitude and Appreciation*: The expression of gratitude and appreciation is also an important component of a Positive Mindset. Gratitude has been described by Froh and Bono (2011, p. 1) *as* 'a higher-level moral emotion that enables people to notice, understand and capitalise on beneficial exchanges with others'. It has been described as the most important cohesive element for an effective functioning society (Simmel 1996). Gratitude has two components:

- Acknowledging the supportive or generous actions of others towards you and expressing thanks to those responsible (Emmons 2007).
- Feeling grateful for the good things in your own day-to-day life and life in the bigger picture. Howells (2012) refers to gratitude as an inner attitude that can be understood as the opposite of resentment or complaint (Howells 2012).

In a study by Froh et al. (2008), young adolescents (aged 11–14) took part in an educational curriculum intervention in which they were asked to undertake a daily routine for two weeks in which they identified 5 things in their life for which they were grateful. These participants, in comparison to a similar group of same-age adolescents who did not participate in the intervention, were assessed three weeks after the intervention as being happier, more optimistic, and more satisfied with their school, family, community, friends, and themselves. They also gave more emotional support to other people in their life. There was also evidence that the gratitude intervention was linked to enhanced psychological and social functioning up to 6 months later (Froh et al. 2010).

There are many strategies that can be employed to teach and encourage students, teachers and other members of the school community to feel and express gratitude. However if gratitude exercises become inauthentic and not a genuine expression of a person's deep-felt 'attitude of gratitude' then the exercise is self-defeating.

- Very young children can begin to learn about gratitude if they are taught to notice the help or support others such as their teacher, parent-helper or another student or older buddy-helper have offered in some way and learn to say thanks. As children move through primary school they increasingly become capable of making accurate judgments about when an adult or another student is being generous or supportive towards them without advantage and at some cost to themselves (Froh and Bono 2011; Emmons and Shelton 2002).
- A 'Gratitude Bulletin Board' can be located in classrooms, school hallways, school dining rooms and in the staff room on which people are encouraged to write down the things they are grateful for about the school and its members.
- A 'Thank you' board placed in the staffroom specifically encourages staff to express their appreciation for support given by their colleagues.
- A regular time each week can be set aside for students to write in their 'Gratitude Journal'
- An 'Appreciation Station' strategy (McGrath and Noble 2011a, b) can be used as a weekly gratitude activity. This requires a specific area in the classroom or a shared general purpose room where a class of students can be given time to write cards or letters to genuinely express their appreciation and gratitude to someone. The activity can be linked with English, art and craft and design and technology (e.g. making a pop-up card)
- Each student in a class can be asked to contribute one page each term to the creation of a 'Digital Classroom Gratitude Book' book. They are asked to keep notes throughout each term of things they are grateful for in their day-to-day lives as well as the kind and supportive behaviour by others that they have appreciated
- Howells (2012) refers to the 'butterfly effect' of teachers' small gratitude practices with their students and parents that can have a transformational effect, especially on difficult students or parents. These practices may include saying thank you, greeting others by smiling or waving at them, looking for the good in others, sending notes of thanks or reflecting on what they are grateful for in their students on the way to work.

(vi) *Mindfulness* In positive psychology there is increasing interest in the benefits of mindfulness and acceptance for mental health and wellbeing. Mindfulness has been described as the self-regulation of attention with the use of an attitude of curiosity, openness and acceptance (Bishop et al. 2004). It means paying attention to the present moment without judgement (Niemiec 2014). In contrast being on 'auto pilot' can mean people are less aware of what is happening. This can mean they miss the details (often positives) of life and also miss opportunities to grow or challenge themselves (Niemiec 2014). Fredrickson et al. (2008) found the mindfulness practice of loving-kindness meditation produced increases over time in daily experiences of positive emotions that, in turn, increased personal resources (e.g. purpose in life, social support). A review of 14 studies integrating mindfulness training in schools found the following student improvements: social skills, academic skills, emotional regulation, self esteem, positive mood and academic skills and better memory and attention. Students also showed less anxiety, stress and fatigue (Meiklejohn et al. 2012).

Practising mindfulness. Niemiec (2014) refers to three ways in which mindfulness may be practised

- *Formally*: In this approach a certain time each day or each week is allocated for students to use mindfulness techniques. Niemiec (2014) suggests a maximum of 10 min per day for children (Niemiec 2014). The most common form is encouraging students to concentrate on their breathing. The Smiling Mind app http://smilingmind.com.au has free mindfulness scripts for age 7–11 years, 12–15 years and 16–22 years. A walking meditation where children walk in silence through a park or garden or similar attractive area in one or two long lines following each other can work well with young children up to ten years of age.
- *Informally*: In this approach students are encouraged to practise mindfulness when they need to calm down i.e. '*use it when you need it*'. This may occur when students are feeling anxious, overwhelmed or depressed and the teacher encourages them to slow down, pause and 'just be'. The teacher can assist them to breathe deeply, and become aware of their body, their feelings, their behaviour and their environment. They can also be encouraged to think about how they can help themselves feel better.
- *In-the-moment approach*: Students are encouraged to return to the present moment whenever their mind wanders and do one thing at a time rather than multi-task. They can also be encouraged to pay full attention to what they are currently doing (*in terms of seeing, hearing, smelling and touching*) and to practise 'being' in the present.

(vii) *Savouring* is a term that describes intentionally intensifying and prolonging a pleasurable experience or feeling by thinking deeply about the positive feelings and sensations involved. It can also encourage mindfulness. Students can be taught to savour small experiences at school or at home or focus in this way on past experiences and positive emotions or future eagerly anticipated experiences. They can do this through thinking, writing, drawing or explaining their experiences to other people. The following examples apply four 'savouring' strategies (suggested by Bryant and Veroff (2007) to the classroom context.

(a) *Savouring by sharing experiences with other people*: At the end of each day, several students can be selected to share (e.g. in small groups or in whole-class Circle Time) one thing they enjoyed the most about the day or the previous weekend/school holiday, one new thing they did in class that really interested them etc. The teacher can use prompting questions such as: What did it feel like? Why did you enjoy it so much? What was the best part of it for you?

(b) *Memory-Building*: students can be asked to create mental photographs of a positive event that they recently took part in such as an excursion or a performance that they saw or participated in. These positive reconstructions can be supported by photographs, souvenirs from the event such as a toy dinosaur from the museum or a shell from a visit to the beach. Two picture books for young primary aged children that promote the development of positive memory-building are *Good Mood Hunt* by Hiawyn Oram and Joanne Partis and *Wilfred Gordon McDonald Partridge* by Mem Fox and Julie Vivas. A useful picture book for older students is *The Secret of Saying Thanks* by Douglas Wood and Greg Shed.

(c) *Self-Congratulation*: Providing opportunities in class time or school assemblies for students to share their achievements allows them to savour the achievement and savour associated positive emotions such as satisfaction and pride.

(d) *Sharpening Sensory-Perceptions*: Students can be encouraged to be more attentive to what they are experiencing by asking them to specifically focus on what they are seeing, smelling, tasting, hearing and feeling. They can also be asked to write a gratitude poem about, for example the beach, writing one line for each sense (I see, I hear, I smell, I feel, I taste, I am thankful for) (McGrath and Noble 2011a, b). Here is an example of such a poem written by a 14 year-old student

> *Sun glistening on water*
> *Waves crash on the sand*
> *The air smells of seaweed*
> *Water rushes through my hand*
> *My fingers taste of salt*
> *I love the beach*

A 'wonder wand' activity (McGrath and Noble 2011a, b) can also be used as a strategy for helping younger students to sharpen their sensory perceptions and sense of 'awe'. Each child makes a wonder wand (a stick with a star on the end works well) which they use to touch or point at things they see on a class walk around the school playground or the local park and ask 'wonder 'questions such as 'I wonder why most of the flowers we saw are bright colours, I wonder why the roses smelled so nice'. These sensory perceptions are then followed up in a classroom activity where they draw and write about what they saw and research answers to some of the questions asked on their walk.

2.3   PROSPER Pathway 2.: Building Positive RELATIONSHIPS

2.3.1   Positive School Culture

Schools are complex social environments. The culture of a school impacts on everyone in the school community: students, the school leadership team, the teachers and families. The contribution of positive relationships to student well-being and learning and to the development of a positive, safe, supportive and connected school culture is a significant and recurring theme in research studies. A positive school culture is characterised by positive student peer relationships, positive student–teacher relationships, positive staff relationships and positive family-school relationships. The intentional development of these relationships is the starting point not only for a positive school culture but also enhanced student engagement and success in learning (Cohen et al. 2010; Battistich 2001; Battistich et al. 1995; Benard 2004; Resnick et al. 1997).

The terms school culture and school climate are often used interchangeably. School climate refers to the quality and character of school life. School climate is defined by the US National School Climate Center as patterns of people's experiences of school life and reflects a school's norms, goals, values, interpersonal relationships, teaching and learning practices, and organizational structures (Thapa et al. 2012). In their document titled the *Foundation for Democracy: Promoting Social, Emotional, Ethical, Cognitive Skills and Dispositions in K-12 Schools*, Cohen et al. (2010) argued that measuring and working to improve school climate is the single most powerful K-12 educational strategy that supports a school to intentionally create a positive school community. Such communities develop the skills, knowledge and dispositions that support student wellbeing and their capacity to learn and become engaged and effective citizens. Researchers such as O'Malley et al. (2012) and Cohen et al's (2010) review of empirical research literature indicated that a positive school climate is associated with/or predictive of academic achievement, school success, effective violence prevention, students' healthy development and teacher retention.

A study by McGrath et al. (2005) highlighted the importance of taking a positive psychology approach to the issues of school bullying. Eleven schools (6 primary and 5 secondary) with relatively low levels of bullying were identified in an attempt to look at 'what works' in reducing bullying rather than 'what goes wrong'. Data were collected through one-to-one interviews with school leaders, observations, focus group inter-views with students, teachers and parents and an analysis of these schools' policies and school curriculum documents. Through a thematic analysis of the data, four positive factors emerged as having the strongest impact on (i) building a safe and supportive school culture and (ii) keeping levels of bullying low. These four factors were:

1. Making student wellbeing a high priority in the school
2. Having a school leadership team who empowered and worked effectively with key teachers and the whole staff to develop (or continue) a whole school vision based around the safety, wellbeing and personal growth of students
3. Having a whole-school positive behaviour management program in place that was working well (*even though no two schools had exactly the same behaviour management approach*)
4. Planning for a 'relationship culture' that focused on the intentional development of positive peer relationships through the adoption of strategies such as cooperative learning, explicit teaching of social skills and pro-social values, cross-age sporting and drama activities and lunchtime clubs

These four factors offer direction to school leadership. A clear message from this research is the importance of a whole school focus on student wellbeing and the intentional development of a safe, supportive and connected school culture.

This section reviews how a safe and supportive school culture is underpinned by a school's pro-social values and how these values are demonstrated through successful positive relationships.

Endorsing and promoting positive values A school's values are intrinsic to all that a school does. A starting point in building a safe, supportive, respectful and connected school culture is for a school community to clarify and reach agreement about the values that will guide their school's practices. If a school articulates pro-social values through it's vision statement, policies, structures and teaching practices, then these values help to form a 'moral map' that helps everyone in the school community to make positive choices about how they interact with each other

The importance of a school's practice in articulating their school values to guide the development of a safe and supportive school culture is illustrated in the large-scale values education project funded by the Australian Government (Lovat and Toomey 2007). The Values Education Project involved 166 schools in 26 school clusters and 70,000 students. The starting point for many schools in this Values Project was helping their school community to clarify and reach agreement about the values that would guide their school's practices (Lovat and Toomey 2007). A key outcome from the project was the recognition by everyone in the school community that their wellbeing was derived from contributing to the wellbeing of others. The project's final report observed that '*involving more people in the enterprise takes more time but ensures deeper commitment, stronger consistency and durable continuity beyond personnel changes*'. (Implementing the National Framework for Values Education in Australian Schools: Final Report 2006, p. 2)

What are the values that resonate across cultures and are universally acceptable to both individualistic Western cultures as well as collectivist cultures of Africa, Asia and the Middle East? According to the former President of UNESCO, Lourdes Quisumbling values are an integral component of education and are essential if an individual is to 'survive, to live and work in dignity and to continue learning'. The values Quisumbling identifies for personal and social transformation are: peace, human rights, dignity, democracy, tolerance, justice, cooperation and sustainable development. From surveys of more than 25,000 people in 44 countries, Schwartz (2011) identified ten types of universal values. These values fall on two dimensions: self-transcendence (i.e. *more concerned with collective interests*) and self-enhancement (i.e. *more concerned with individual interests*).

- *Self-enhancement* (individualism) is represented by nine values in Schwartz' research: social power, wealth, social recognition, authority, self-respect, ambition, influence, capability and success.
- *Self-transcendence* (collectivism) is represented by fifteen values: equality, a world at peace, unity with nature, wisdom, a world of beauty, social justice, broadmindedness, a protected environment, mature love, true friendship, loyalty, honesty, helpfulness, responsibility and forgiveness.

Of relevance to education contexts that support student wellbeing, people who give priority to self-transcendent values are more willing to engage in altruistic, cooperative and/or ecologically responsible behaviour that underpins the development of positive relationships than people who give priority to individual or self-enhancement values (Schwartz 2011).

Teaching values: How can self-transcendent values that accord with student wellbeing be readily communicated to children and young people in schools to effectively guide their behaviour? Several studies have linked the direct teaching of pro-social values with improved academic and social outcomes in schools (e.g. Lovat and Toomey 2007; Zins et al. 2004; Benninga et al. 2003; Battistich et al. 2001). 'Values education' initiatives in schools have been shown to extend the strategies, options and repertoires of teachers in effectively managing learning environments and in developing supportive and connected school and class cultures that positively connect learners with their classmates and teachers (Lovat and Clement 2008; Carr 2006). A focus on values has also been shown to increase students' sense of safety from bullying and harassment (Battistich et al. 2001; Cowie and Olafsson 2000; Cross et al. 2004; Flannery et al. 2003). From their experience in working with schools implementing the Australian Framework in Values Education, Lovat and Toomey (2007) concluded that values education is at the heart of quality teaching.

A whole school approach to defining and teaching values to guide behaviour is also the starting point for the highly successful model of School-wide Positive Behavior Support (SWPBS). The purpose of SWPBS is to first establish a school climate based on positive values so that they become the norm. Typically each school chooses 3–5 values that can also become behavioural expectations. An example of this is the value of 'respect' which can then become expectations such as '*Respect Yourself, Respect Others and Respect Property*'. The SWPBS guidelines highlight the importance of at least 80 % of the staff making a commitment to the school's chosen values defined as behavioural expectations in order to ensure there is consistency in implementation from class to class (https://www.pbis.org/school/swpbis-for-beginners) To facilitate consistency across the school, it is suggested that each school develops an 'expectations matrix' of what the values in action look like in all

Table 2.2 An expectations matrix

School setting	Safe	Respectful	Learner
Formal occasions	• Follow staff directions	• Be quiet, respectful and courteous	• Participate as required
	• Enter and exit in an orderly manner	• Use acceptable language, tone and voice	
Sport	• Play by the rules	• Wear correct uniform	• Actively participate
	• Use equipment safely	• Play fair	• Be positive
	• Stay with your teacher	• Be a good sportsperson	• Be respectful
Learning space	• Be on time	• Be ready to learn	• Be a good listener
	• Follow classroom rules and expectation	• Allow students to learn	• Do your best
	• Use equipment safely	• Allow teachers to teach	• Take responsibility for your learning
Corridors/transition/bus	• Walk safely	• Keep area clean	• Be respectful
	• Stay on your left	• Go straight to class	• Be safe
	• Move quietly	• Keep hands and feet to self	• Be on time
Playground	• Follow directions	• Respect others	• Report incidents
	• Stay in bounds	• Respect the environment	• Go to class on time
Toilets/canteen	• Walk	• Wait for turn	• Use good manners
	• Wash hand	• Be polite	• Keep the area clean
	• Go straight to class	• Save water	• Use bins

classes and non-classroom areas (see Table 2.2). Teaching behavioural expectations based on pro-social values and rewarding students for following them has been found to be a much more positive and preventative approach than waiting for misbehaviors to occur before responding. SWPBS is a set of intervention practices and organisational systems for establishing a positive school culture and intensive individual behaviour supports to achieve academic and social success for all students (Sugai et al. 2009). Multiple randomized control trials have documented improvement in student outcomes when SWPBS is implemented (e.g., Bradshaw et al. 2008, 2009; Horner et al. 2009). The following table provides an example of a large secondary school's expectations matrix developed in conjunction with staff and students. The matrix is displayed in every classroom, hallway and formal spaces.

The Australian Values Education Good Practice Schools Projects Implementing the National Framework for Values Education in Australian Schools: Final Report

(2006), found that effective values education is more likely to occur when a school's shared values are explicitly articulated, explicitly taught, modelled by staff and embedded in the mainstream life of the school. This means values education is most effective when it is integrated in the mainstream curriculum rather than being an 'add-on' or separate to the academic curriculum. It also means that teachers consciously create many opportunities for students to practise the values. The values most likely to be included in school—based values programs are: *Compassion, Cooperation, Acceptance of difference, Respect, Friendliness/ Inclusion, Honesty, Fairness and Responsibility* (McGrath and Noble 2011a, b). These core values have been taught to both young and older children through the use of children's literature, media stories, video-clips, role-plays, writing activities and opportunities for students to engage in classroom and school community activities that provide service to others.

- *Compassion*: Caring about the wellbeing of others and offering kindness and support where needed;
- *Cooperation*: Working together to achieve a shared goal. Cooperating also includes cooperating for world peace and for the protection of our environment;
- *Acceptance of differences*: Recognising the right of others to be different and not excluding or mistreating others because they are different; acting on the inclusive belief that diversity is to be celebrated and other people are fundamentally good;
- *Respect for others*: Acting towards others in ways that respect their rights; for example to have dignity, to have their feelings considered, to be safe and to be treated fairly;
- *Friendliness*: Acting towards others in an inclusive and kind way; actively reaching out to others in friendship
- *Honesty*: Telling the truth, and owning up to anything you have done;
- *Fairness*: Focusing on equity and addressing injustices; and
- *Responsibility*: Acting in ways that honour promises and commitments and looking after the wellbeing of those less able.

Case Study

Values in action across the school

When we met Gerda v d Westhuizen she was the principal of the Observatory School for Girls, a school in a very impoverished area of Johannesburg where many families were refugees from other African countries, where often four families shared one room, and where there was no hope of work for most of these families who were just surviving. Gerda's explicit focus on values formed the core business of the whole school community. She chose one of the twelve values from the UNESCO's *Living Values* program every two weeks to become the central focus for everyone's work and behaviour across the school. The twelve Living Values are freedom, cooperation, tolerance, happiness, honesty, love, peace, humility, respect, responsibility, simplicity, and unity. Gerda drew the children's attention to the school's current 'value' by making a visually stimulating and eye-catching display of the value and especially the actions the students could take to put that value into action. This display was on a notice board in a prominent place in the school playground. The most highly prized award in the school was the opportunity that a student from every class at each grade level had to wear the values gold sash award for a week that showed that this student had been observed putting this value into action through their interactions with others across the school.

Respectful language can change school culture

Values education is also at the heart of one secondary school's approach to how language used in communication between students and teachers or between different students can be inclusive or exclusive. In a large Australian state government secondary school for boys all teaching staff were united in encouraging all the boys to use language that is inclusive of everyone. The staff noticed and reprimanded any boy who used negative language that was homophobic, racist, sexist or in any way was derogatory and served through what people said to each other to exclude certain individuals or groups from the school community. The principal reported that this one small action has had a huge impact on making their school a safer and supportive school community. The interview with the school principal can be seen at http://www.safeschoolshub.edu.au/safe-schools-toolkit/the-nine-elements/element-5/case-studies/melbourne-hs-element-5/.

Values captains

Many schools have school captains but one primary school appointed two Values captains as well as two School captains. Values Captains helped the whole school community focus on noticing their values in action. A poster of the school's values was displayed in every classroom, hallways and staff room. Every two weeks the Values Captains gave out Values certificates in Assembly to those children who had being observed demonstrating one of the school's values. For example a student is awarded a certificate for Honesty because they handed into the office money they had found in the playground.

2.3.2   Building Positive Student-Peer Relationships

When students act in accord with pro-social values such as being friendly and inclusive, respectful of others and supportive, compassionate and kind, then they are more likely to develop positive and satisfying relationships with both their teachers and their peers. Students who experience predominantly positive and high quality peer relationships at school are more likely to experience better mental and physical health, improved learning outcomes and more successful relationships as adults (Engels et al. 2001; Rhodes et al. 2000). Positive peer relationships are also linked to higher levels of attendance at school, high levels of engagement with schoolwork and a higher likelihood of finishing high school.

Friendships are a significant source of emotional and psychological support for students and contribute to their sense of belonging (La Greca and Harrison 2005). Friendships can provide students with closeness, a sense of connection and safety, affirmation and, when needed, social and practical support. Friendships also provide a context in which students can practise and refine their social skills and develop empathy and socio-moral reasoning. (Hodges et al. 1999; Schonert-Reichl 1999; Thoma and Ladewig 1993). Students who experience considerable social isolation, or who are not well accepted or are actively rejected are less likely to be engaged with learning, and are more likely to be absent from school and have poorer learning outcomes and a reduced sense of wellbeing (e.g. Ladd 2003; Ladd and Burgess 2001; Marks 2000; Ladd et al. 1997; Boivin et al. 1995; Hatzichristou and Hopf 1996; Ollendick et al. 1992). Students who are chronically socially isolated or rejected are also more likely, as adults, to have less satisfactory and successful lives and be more likely to experience depression, erratic employment and involvement with crime (McDougall et al. 2001; Blackorby and Wagner 1996; Gresham 1986). Students who have poor relationships with peers are also more likely to use drugs, misbehave, report anxiety/depressive symptoms, and drop out before finishing high school (Bond et al. 2007; Doll and Hess 2001; Marcus and Sanders-Reio 2001; Barclay and Doll 2001; Resnick et al. 1997; Catalano et al. 1996). A student's level of social competence and their friendship networks have been shown to be predictive of their level of academic achievement (Caprara et al. 2000; Wentzel and Caldwell 1997). A study found that 3rd grade children's social competence predicted their grades in 8th grade better than their academic performance in 3rd grade (Caprara et al. 2000). A meta-analysis of 148 studies involving 17,000 students conducted in 11 different countries concluded that positive peer relationships explained 33–40 % of variation in academic achievement (Roseth et al. 2008).

Criss et al. (2002) have demonstrated that being accepted by peers and having friends can moderate aggressive and acting-out behaviour in young children with disadvantaged family backgrounds characterised by economic difficulties, family violence and harsh discipline. Research also suggests that having at least one best friend can help prevent children and young people from being bullied (Bollmer et al. 2005). However the number of friendships that a child has is less important than the quality of those friendships. In their study Werner and Smith (1992) identified that resilient young people were not necessarily popular or very well accepted but had developed a small number of high quality, long-lasting friendships characterised by loyalty and support. High quality friendships are characterised by this kind of loyalty and support as well as a willingness to stand up for their friend (Bollmer et al. 2005). In contrast, poor quality friendships are associated with negative characteristics such as conflict or betrayal and, in some cases, with being bullied (Greco and Morris 2005; Mishima 2003; Mishna et al. 2008). It seems likely that the positive effects of school-based relationships are probably the result of a student's cumulative experience of such reciprocated friendships over time rather than the result of specific individual friendships (Hartup and Stevens 1997).

One way schools develop positive student-peer relationships across year levels is through the implementation of peer support programs. Stanley and Mcgrath (2006) conducted an investigation in 12 schools into the perceptions held by primary teachers and senior staff of the advantages they had observed from their experiences of using a 'buddy system' in which every child in the first two years of school (ages 5–6 years) had an older student (aged 11–12 years) as a 'special friend'. The advantages that were identified included that they helped build positive relationships and connectedness across the school, helped the younger students to experience a sense of belonging and feel supported and safe, and assisted the older students to develop responsibility, confidence, leadership behaviours and social skills. Several studies (e.g. Menesini et al. 2003) have identified that teachers report that their school environment becomes safer and more caring following the introduction of a befriending scheme, and that peer relationships across the school improve.

2.3.2.1 Teaching the Social–Emotional Skills that Underpin Positive Peer Relationships

Research indicates that there are potentially many positive outcomes from proactively and explicitly teaching students the following social and emotional skills (McGrath and Francey 1991; McGrath and Noble 2010, 2011a, b) and pro-social values that have the power to facilitate positive peer relationships.

- *Specific Social skills*: The key social skills that are related to both learning activities and out-of-class interpersonal interactions are skills for: sharing resources and workload (i.e. cooperation), respectfully disagreeing (*stating points of agreement before explaining where you disagree*), negotiation, playing fairly, responding empathically, having an interesting conversation, presenting to an audience, telling a funny story or joke, and managing conflict well. Social skills are not only 'relationship builders' but are also 'academic enablers' (Wentzel and Caldwell 1997; Wentzel and Watkins 2002)
- *Emotional literacy skills*: These include skills for managing strong feelings such as anger, fear and disappointment and skills for recognising and understanding the feelings of others and responding empathically.

Embedding the teaching and practice of these skills within the curriculum pro-vides naturalistic opportunities for students to practise these skills once they have been explicitly taught.

The following section illustrates how (i) cooperative learning, (ii) cooperative games and (iii) using children's literature can assist teachers to embed the teaching of social skills into the curriculum and build positive peer relationships.

(i) *Using Cooperative Learning to teach and enable practice of Social-emotional Skills.*

The use of cooperative learning structures creates opportunities for teachers to actively engage students in a curriculum activity whilst at the same time providing naturalistic situations for them to practise social skills and access peer support for their learning. The numerous research outcomes for cooperative learning can be organized under three broad categories: improving student *effort to achieve; building positive relationships and support;* and *enhancing student wellbeing* (Johnson and Johnson 2009). Roseth et al. (2008) carried out a meta-analysis of 148 studies that compared the impact of cooperative, competitive, and individualistic learning activities on adolescent students. They found that the use of cooperative group structures had the most impact on academic achievement and positive peer relationships. Similar conclusions were reached in earlier studies that linked peer learning methods to better social outcomes (e.g. Ginsburg-Block et al. 2006).

Cooperative learning structures promote positive social interactions that are associated with mutual assistance, encouragement of each other and the sharing of ideas, information and resources that contribute to the achievement of shared goals. The achievement of these collaborative goals enhances the likelihood that students will develop positive perceptions of each other and the contributions each group member made to group success (Roseth et al. 2008). This process also creates a sense of belonging that helps to facilitate student engagement and other adaptive school behaviors (Juvonen 2006). The essential principles of cooperative learning that are the key to achieving these outcomes are:

- the structure of the group learning ensures there is individual accountability and everyone 'pulls their weight' rather than leaving the hard work to just one or two people
- there is group interdependence in that everyone is responsible for both their own and their group's learning outcomes, and
- social skills (e.g. *listening, turn taking, sharing the workload and the discussion space, negotiating, respectful disagreeing*) are explicitly taught and then prac-tised in the group work.

A reflection sheet that can be completed by the group as a whole can be helpful in identifying the social skills that each group member used well or needed to use more (e.g. see McGrath and Noble 2010).

(ii) *Using Cooperative Games to teach social-emotional skills.*

Most students find playing games (whether they are physical or educational games) engaging, motivating and fun. When students play games together they have an opportunity to experience positive emotions such as excitement and enjoyment as well as opportunities to socially interact with classmates, practise emotional skills (e.g. *self regulation of anger and aggression*) and practise social skills (e.g. *conflict management, playing fairly and being a good winner/loser*) within a naturally occurring social context. Additionally, many educational games such as quizzes have the potential to reinforce curriculum content and provide opportunities for deductive reasoning and other higher order thinking skills (e.g. McGrath and Noble 2010). Hill (1989) has pointed out that structured co-operative games and tasks provide opportunities for more popular children to interact with lower status peers who they may choose to avoid in other situations. Through playing cooperative class games, the more popular children can get to know the other children and experience success with their less popular peers.

The rules and procedures that are a core part of any game provide both structure and limits. These features make it more likely that students will behave more pro-socially and less aggressively when playing educational games (Garaigardobil et al. 1996). It can also be useful to include a briefing session at the start of the game in which the rules and expected social skills that will make the game more successful and fun are highlighted and discussed (McGrath and Francey 1991; McGrath and Noble 2010). The 'Educational Games Tournament structure' (McGrath and Noble 2010, 2011a, b) is an additional feature that can further enhance the impact of practising social and emotional skills and the development of positive relationships. In this structure, students work with a partner to play (as a pair) a specific educational game (e.g. Hangman-see McGrath and Noble 2010 for other suggestions) against five different student pairs over a week or so. Pairs stay the same for the duration of the tournament (usually just one week) thus having a chance to get to know each other a bit better and to improve their game strategies and social skills. Over time, all students can have an opportunity to play in a partnership with every other student in the class. Each pair can complete a self-assessment rubric after the tournament has been completed, rating themselves on how well they (as a pair) used good thinking strategies, how effectively they set improvement goals and how well they used social skills such as listening to each other, managing conflict well, playing fairly, respectful disagreeing, winning and losing well, negotiation and respecting the effort of all players. The teacher can then conduct a Debriefing session after the tournament to revise and reinforce the social skills that were highlighted in the briefing session at the start of the tournament.

Cooperative games can also provide a naturalistic setting in which to conduct an assessment of the social and emotional skills of specific students. This can be the basis for further more intensive teaching of specific social skills in small group contexts.

(iii) *Using children's literature to teach social-emotional skills.*

Another strategy for embedding social-emotional learning in the curriculum is through the use of good quality children's literature. All countries have stories such as myths, legends, and fairytales that can teach children key messages about wellbeing and resilience. Infusing the teaching of social and emotional skills into the academic curriculum through picture books and stories and follow-up classroom discussions enables students to further increase their understanding of relationships and how to manage them.

Books can start conversations. According to Phillips (2008, p. 2) *"a well told story invites listeners to enter the world of the story, identify with the characters and accompany them on the journey of experience, then emerge with new insight and understandings"*. Through books, students can engage with key real life issues such as friendships in a safe and comfortable way and a teacher can choose a book with relevance for one student or a group without specifically focusing on them. Students are able to discuss a problem that is linked to a book's character without owning that problem. Books can also 'normalise' a situation such as loneliness and help a student to realise that they are not the first or only person to encounter such a problem. Students can also feel and express empathy for a character in a specific situation and this can enhance their empathy for 'real people' in a similar situation. Books can prompt self-reflection and insight. A character in a book can be used as a positive model when they display a pro-social value such as kindness, solve a relationship problem through the use of a social skill such as negotiation or get on top of a situation by using an emotional skill such as managing their anger or being courageous. The use of books in this way is dependent on the quality of the book itself and the knowledge and insight of the author and illustrator. Gruwell and Freedom Writers (1999) provided powerful examples of how helping under-privileged high school students relate their life troubles to literary stories and social values can have dramatic positive effects on their engagement with school.

The use of children's literature to teach students about wellbeing and resilience was at the heart of the Bushfire Recovery Project by the Victorian Education Department (McGrath and Noble 2011b). In 2009 the Australian state of Victoria experienced the worst bushfires in the history of Australia with great loss of life, homes and whole communities. The Victorian Education Department implemented the Bounce Back Wellbeing and Resilience Program in seven regions affected by these devastating fires. Every school in the project was given a tub of forty picture books to support the implementation of the program. Findings from the implementation of Bounce Back over two school terms in 18 schools affected by the Victorian bushfires yielded 11 themes. The key themes emerged from the integration of data from an online teacher survey with focus group discussions in six schools with both teachers and children. The data showed that the Bounce Back lessons helped the children to cope better and be resilient with the aftermath of the bushfires. The teachers saw the use of children's literature as one of the strongest and most important features of the implementation. The following comments illustrate the teachers' enthusiasm for their use of children's literature: *The books helped the children to discuss problems more freely; I have certainly used the books with students to encourage more positive/helpful thinking; The books have been terrific as they in some cases take the focus off particular children while addressing class or individual problems.*

2.3.3   Building Positive Student–Teacher Relationships

Students' perception that their teachers care about them is among the strongest predictors of student performance (Dweck et al. 2015). Having a relationship with a caring adult other than, or in addition to, a parent has been shown to be a significant protective factor in helping young people to be resilient (Garmezy 1991). This person is often a teacher (Benard 2004). Hence it is perceived as the professional responsibility of teachers to be proactive in developing a positive relationship with each of their students (Krause et al. 2006; Marzano 2003: McInerney and McInerney 2006).

The quality of students' relationships with their teachers strongly influences how they feel about and respond to school and their schoolwork. Most students want their teachers to like and care about them and look for signs that this is or isn't the case. Positive high quality teacher–student relationships are characterised, depending on the age of the student, by many of the following features (e.g. Battistich et al. 2004; Hamre and Pianta 2001):

- Low levels of teacher–student conflict
- Low levels of student dependency
- High levels of mutually respectful behaviour
- Teacher acceptance, warmth, caring and closeness and predictability
- High levels of teacher support for the student

When students perceive that they have this type of relationship with their teacher (s) they feel more secure and hence are more willing to engage with learning activities and the school environment (Baumeister and Leary 1995; Deci and Ryan 1985; Furrer and Skinner 2003; Roorda et al. 2011). They are also more likely to have high rates of school attendance, (Klem and Connell 2004), demonstrate high levels of achievement motivation and academic effort and, at the high school level, to commit to finishing their schooling (e.g. Hattie 2009; Klem and Connell 2004; Martin et al. 2007; Marzano et al. 2003; Roorda et al. 2011) and achieve more highly (Battistich et al. 2004; Hamre and Pianta 2001). These patterns are illustrated in a comprehensive study of 3450 students in years 7–12 across six Australian high schools (Martin et al. 2007). Those students who believed that their teacher accepted and cared for them, were more engaged with learning, felt more confident and motivated to achieve and were more likely to adopt the teacher's goals and expectations in relation to school success.

Other positive student outcomes that have been identified as associated with caring and supportive teacher–student relationships include higher levels of academic resilience, social competency and overall wellbeing (Battistich et al. 2004; Howes and Ritchie 1999; Nadel and Muir 2005; Pianta et al. 2008; Pianta and

Walsh 1996; Raskauskas et al. 2010; Weare 2000). Feeling supported and cared for by teachers is also protective against bullying and being bullied (Flashpohler et al. 2009). Resnick et al. (1997), found that young people who reported having a close and positive relationship with their teachers were less likely to use drugs and alcohol, attempt suicide or self-harm, behave in violent ways or engage in sexual behaviour at an early age.

A study by Hughes et al. (2001) suggested that when teachers take the trouble to develop a positive relationship with socially vulnerable students, they make it more likely that other students will behave towards them in a more socially inclusive way. The quality of teacher–student relationships also impacts on the effectiveness of a teacher's classroom management. In their meta-analysis of research studies, Marzano et al. (2003) found that, on average, teachers who had high-quality relationships with their students had 31 % fewer discipline and related problems in a given year than teachers who did not have this type of relationship with their students. This is well explained by students who experience such relationships with their teacher being more open and responsive to their directions and advice (Gregory et al. 2010), more reluctant to disappoint them by behaving badly or engaging in anti-social behaviour such as bullying, and being more comfortable with adopting the values and norms endorsed by their teachers and their school (Bergin and Bergin 2009; Masten and Obradović 2008; Stipek 2006).

When evaluating whether or not their teacher is a 'good' teacher', students tend to focus most on the interpersonal quality of their relationship with them (Rowe 2004; Slade and Trent 2000; Werner 2002). Some of the components of positive and supportive teacher–student relationships may vary according to the age of the student and the level of involvement of the teacher, but the following teacher behaviours have been identified by either students, teachers or both as contributing to positive student-teacher relationships:

• Teachers acknowledge students, greet them by name and with a smile and they notice when the students are absent from school and follow up (Benard 1991; Stipek 2006)
• Teachers respond to misbehaviour or inattention with reminders and explanations rather than irritability, criticism, punishment or coercion (Bergin and Bergin 2009; Noddings 1992; Rimm-Kaufman 2011)
• Teachers take a personal interest in their students as individuals and get to know them both as students (Marzano 2003; Stipek 2006; Trent 2001) as well as people with a life outside school (Trent 2001). They demonstrate knowledge about individual students' backgrounds, interests, strengths and academic levels. They strive to understand what each student needs to succeed in school and work with them towards that goal (Croninger and Lee 2001)
• Teachers are available and approachable when students need support or just answers to questions (Pianta 1999; Weissberg et al. 1991) and they take the time to listen to their students when they have concerns or worries and offer support in a timely manner where appropriate (Benard 2004)
• Teachers are fair and respectful when talking to students (Stipek 2006). Keddie and Churchill (2003) found that, when adolescent boys were asked what they

liked about the good relationships they had with certain teachers, they most often referred to the fair and respectful way in which these teachers had spoken to them and treated them.

- Teachers show their pleasure and enjoyment in being with their students and have fun with them when appropriate. They let students get to know them through some degree of self-disclosure and being 'authentic' with them (Davis 2003). In this way common interests and experiences can be identified and bonds start to form.
- Teachers use many learner-centered practices in their teaching (Cornelius-White 2007; Gurland and Grolnick 2003) such as showing sensitivity to individual differences among students, supporting them in the development of autonomy (e.g. by offering them choices and opportunities to be involved in decision-making), respecting and incorporating their views and ideas and noticing, acknowledging and addressing their individual developmental, personal and social needs. They differentiate learning to accommodate student differences and try to spend some individual time with each student (Pianta 1999; Rudasill et al. 2006). They intentionally develop positive peer relationships in a way that ensures that no student feels socially isolated (Charney 2002; Donohue et al. 2003).

Case Study

Buddy programs for whole school positive relationships

The implementation of buddy programs that involve all students and all staff including administration and support staff illustrate one school's focus on the importance of building positive relationships across the whole school community. Like many schools, St Charles Borromeo Primary School in Melbourne for many years has successfully run a buddy program where the year 5 and year 6 children (10–12 year olds) become a buddy for a child (a 5/6 year old) in their first year of school. The buddies connect with each other during informal times in the playground as well as during formal lesson times where the Year six children act as tutors. But St Charles takes the concept of a buddy program further. The years 1/2 children buddy up with the years 3/4 children. Also the school teams up the year 5 children with 'an oldie' at a nearby residential home for elderly people. Once a term (4 times per year) the children and the elderly take turns at hosting a meeting at the residential home or the school and learning from each other. For example the children might teach their elderly buddy about technology such as sending emails etc and the 'oldies' might teach a card game or about their life when they were young. Another variation of the buddy program is that each year 6 child has an adult staff mentor as a buddy who meets their year 6 buddy regularly to prepare them for secondary schooling and early adolescence. Also all new parents/carers are 'buddied up' with existing parents/carers to facilitate the new parents' entry into the school community. In all examples of the school's buddy programs the focus is on reciprocity where both 'buddies' benefit from the positive relationship, gain in-school-community support and value diversity in age, gender, and cultural backgrounds. See an interview with Sue Cahill about the Buddy program at http://www.safeschoolshub.edu.au/safe-schools-toolkit/the-nine-elements/element-2/case-studies/st-charles-ps-element-2/

2.4 PROSPER Pathway 3: Facilitating OUTCOMES

International assessments such as *Trends in International Mathematics and Science Study* (TIMSS), *Programme for International Student Assessment* (PISA) and *Progress in International Reading Literacy Study* (PIRLS) have prompted nations to attach greatest importance on academic outcomes in schools. So it is not surprising that the outcomes that many schools focus on most are those related to academic learning and achievement. School reform initiatives therefore often look to changes in curriculum or pedagogy to improve student learning outcomes. However curriculum and pedagogy are often narrowly defined in terms of academic content and teaching students that content. Yet research on effective teaching and learning shows that this is not the complete picture.

Why do some students perform better than others even when they have the same ability? Research shows that the *psychological factors* encapsulated in PROSPER are critical for achieving positive learning outcomes and ongoing academic success. Students who PROSPER:

- **P**: feel they belong in school socially and academically; they can forgo immediate pleasures for the sake of schoolwork;
- **R**: have positive relationships with their peers and teachers;
- **O**: gain a sense of accomplishment by achieving positive learning outcomes;
- **S**: know their own strengths and limitations and are prepared to work hard;
- **P**: have a sense of purpose in what they are learning at school and it's relevance for their future;
- **E**: are engaged in learning, view effort positively and seek challenging tasks that will help them learn new things rather than tasks in their comfort zone that require little effort but also little opportunity to learn;
- **R**: are resilient and not derailed by difficulty whether intellectual or social. They see a setback as an opportunity for learning or a problem to be solved rather than a failure.

Academic tenacity is a term used by Dweck et al. (2015) to encapsulate the various non-cognitive factors outlined in PROSPER that promote academic learning and achievement. These authors use academic tenacity to refer to the mindsets and skills that allow students to look beyond short-term concerns to longer-term or higher-order goals and to withstand challenges and setbacks to persevere towards these goals. Students' beliefs about their academic ability influence their academic tenacity. Dweck and her colleagues' research found that a central factor in student's academic outcomes was their mindset about their intelligence. Students may view their intelligence as a fixed quantity that they either possess or not (fixed mindset) or a malleable quantity that can be increased with effort and learning (a growth mindset).

Students with a fixed mindset believe their intellectual ability is a limited entity that can lead to destructive thoughts (e.g. *I failed because I'm dumb*), negative feelings (e.g. *humiliated*) and negative behaviour (*giving up*). In contrast students with a growth mindset will often perceive the same challenge or setback as an opportunity to learn. They respond with constructive thoughts (e.g. *maybe I need to change my strategy or try harder*); positive feelings (*excited by the challenge*) and positive behaviour (e.g. *persistence*) (Dweck et al. 2015). What causes these mindsets? Several experimental studies by Dweck and her colleagues (Mueller and Dweck 1998; Blackwell et al. 2007) found that praising students for their ability taught them a fixed mindset (e.g. that's a really high score. You must be smart at these problems). In contrast praising them for their effort or the strategy they used taught them a growth mindset and fostered resilience (e.g. that's a really high score. You must have worked hard at these problems or simply 'that's a really high score').

Students with a fixed mindset tend to focus more on performance goals. For example they endorse performance avoidance goals because they prefer easy work in their comfort zone that helps them to avoid mistakes and setbacks but also creates little opportunities to learn. Students with a growth mindset tend to focus more on mastery goals or learning goals—choosing challenging tasks that could help them learn.

Research also indicates that students are often more motivated and achieve more academic success when classroom activities involve cooperative rather than competitive or individualistic goals (Johnson and Johnson 2009; Roseth et al. 2008). Cooperative learning goals foster a responsibility for your own and your team mates' learning and not wanting to let one's team down. In comparison, in a competitive environment students may be more likely to engage in self-handicapping behaviour by withholding effort so they can attribute their failure to lack of effort rather than lack of ability (Dweck et al. 2015). One student's accomplishment is at another's loss in competitive environments. Not only are competitive environments associated with lower achievement but also students like each other less (Roseth et al. 2008).

Dweck's research on mindset and Baumeister's work (Baumeister and Tierney 2011) on self-control or willpower and Duckworth's research on 'grit' (Duckworth and Seligman 2005) are all seen as factors contributing to academic tenacity. Self-regulatory skills that allow students to stay on task, rise above distractions and navigate obstacles for long-term achievement also contribute to academic tenacity and school achievement. A study by Duckworth and Seligman (2005) found that 8th graders' capacity for self control (assessed by teachers, parents and self-report) was a better predictor of their academic achievement, including their performance on standardised tests, than the students' IQ scores. In fact self control was seen as a better predictor of academic success than their IQ score. Their self control also predicted fewer absences from school, more time spent studying and less time watching television. Given that students encounter more and more distractions in our technology-rich world it is important to understand how to help students turn off distractions so they focus on difficult academic tasks.

Research over the last fifteen years has found that helping people to visualise possible obstacles that might stand in the way of their goals is an important aspect of developing self regulatory skills and achieving outcomes (Oettingen 2014). Oettingen uses the term 'mental contrasting' to describe the process of visualizing potential obstacles. This process involves the following four steps:

- Identify your goal
- Visualise the best possible outcome
- Identify potential obstacles that might get in the way of you achieving this outcome
- Think about each possible obstacle and plan a way to deal with the obstacle if it does occur

Students could also benefit from participating in pairs or in small group or class discussions to identify potential obstacles that might get in their way in relation to goals that many of them have in common such as a delivering an effective class presentation, completing an upcoming assignment or test, putting together a folio of artwork or finding part-time work. Typical obstacles that might be discussed and planned for might include: getting too involved in computer games, family demands, distractions by friends and lack of available time. Duckworth et al. (2011) found that using Oettingen's four step plan increased high school students' efforts to prepare for standardized tests by 60 %. A free app for college students that is based on mental contrasting can be found at: www.woopmylife.org.

Box: Applying the key Outcome messages for success

The WINNERS acronym in the Success unit in the Bounce Back program (McGrath and Noble 2011a, b) incorporates evidence-informed key messages to help students to achieve outcomes and experience a sense of accomplishment. The benefit of an acronym is that it makes it easier for students to remember and recall these key messages.

- What are my strengths (and what is my evidence?)
- Interesting mistakes will happen. (Don't be afraid to make them and learn from them)
- No effort, no results. (No one achieves anything without hard work and self-discipline)
- Never give up (well, hardly ever). See obstacles as problems to be solved and plan ahead.

- Ethics and honesty must be the rule (or it's not worth it)
- Risk-taking is sometimes necessary (but think about it first and be prepared)
- Smart goal setting helps you plan and succeed. (So choose a Specific and Meaningful goal, work out what Actions you need to take, be Realistic and estimate the Time you'll need to do it)

In the Bounce Back program (Book 3, p. 190) students are encouraged to make a *'if-then'* plan by anticipating beforehand what obstacles might stop them from achieving their goal. For example

- *What if you want to finish your project and a friend texts you and wants to come over to your house. Plan what would you say/do?* Or
- *What if your goal is to eat healthier food and less junk food and a friend invites you to McDonalds for their birthday? Plan what you will order before you go.*

Explicitly teaching study skills and self-regulation skills also has the potential to assist students to achieve better academic outcomes. Some of the most effective strategies identified in a meta-analysis study by Lavery (2008) as having a positive impact on learning outcomes included: strategies that organise and transform knowledge (e.g. *by making a plan such as a mindmap or skeleton outline of an assignment*), encouraging students to self evaluate their assignment before submitting it, seeking support through a study partner or group, using a range of strategies to remember key information (e.g. *creating a mnemonic or acronym*) and managing time effectively. Other strategies suggested by Marzano et al. (2001) include helping students to identify similarities and differences, to summarise, and to generate and test hypotheses.

One program titled *The Student Success Skills Program* targeted 5th–9th graders who were below 50th percentile on their state achievement test in reading and maths (Brigman and Webb 2007). The students were taught skills linked to academic tenacity such as: having a growth mindset, learning how to set goals, monitoring their progress and strategies for handling high-pressure situations by learning to breathe deeply and imagine a safe place where they felt supported, protected and in control. Students participating in the program earned higher state test scores in reading and maths than those in the control group. Hattie's (2009) large scale meta-analysis of the in-school and out-of-school factors that contributed to positive learning outcomes highlights the importance of ongoing formative assessment that benefits both teachers and students. Ongoing formative assessment provides students with important feedback on their progress but also provides teachers with regular feedback on how well they are teaching a specific skill or concept so they can adjust their teaching accordingly. Hattie also highlights the importance of providing students with the success criteria for tasks or, preferably, teachers co-developing success criteria with their students. These different strategies show the importance of teachers providing support to students to promote the positive psychological factors that are crucial to students achieving positive learning outcomes at school.

2.5 PROSPER Pathway 4: Focusing on STRENGTHS

Schools that focus on and value the different individual and collective strengths of all members of the school community demonstrate the fourth PROSPER component for sustained student wellbeing. A 'strength' has been defined as ways of behaving, thinking or feeling that an individual has a natural capacity for enjoys doing and which can assist them to achieve optimal functioning while they pursue valued outcomes (Govindji and Linley 2007; Linley and Harrington 2006). A more recent definition by Wood et al. (2011) describes 'personal strengths' as the characteristics of a person that allows them to perform well or at their personal best. Using one's strengths in schoolwork has been found to be far more enjoyable and productive than working on one's weaknesses, especially for those students whose strengths   are   not   in   the   traditional   academic   domain   (Noble   2004). A strengths-based approach does not ignore weaknesses, but rather helps students achieve outcomes by building on their strengths and understanding and managing their limitations. When people work with their strengths they tend to learn more readily, perform at a higher level, are more motivated and confident, and have a stronger sense of satisfaction, mastery and competence (Clifton and Harter 2003; Peterson and Seligman 2004; Linley and Harrington 2006).

A 'strength' can be a specific skill or ability such writing, reading, playing music, swimming, cartooning, leadership or using spread-sheets. It can also be a character trait such as persistence, bravery, kindness to others, sense of humour. Gardner's (1983, 2006) theory of multiple intelligences for ability strengths and Peterson and Seligman's (2004) model for character strengths are both useful frameworks for educators to utilise in school settings and have been applied in class and school settings (e.g. see Kornhaber et al. 2003; McGrath and Noble 2005a, b; McGrath and Noble 2011a, b; Chen et al. 2009; Peterson and Seligman 2004; Yeager et al. 2011).

The first step for teachers in using a strengths-based approach is to help students to select strategies for the identification of their strengths so they have an opportunity to develop a deep understanding of their relative strengths and weaknesses. The second step is to collaboratively design and implement educational programs and environments in which students can first explore and then apply their strengths in a productive and satisfying way. A strengths-based approach also encourages students to understand that any work that does not engage one of their natural strengths may require a lot more effort to develop competency and mastery in the domains tapped by that strength.

2.5.1 *Ability Strengths*

Howard Gardner's (1983, 2006) model of multiple intelligences (MI) provides directions for the identification and development of ability strengths. MI theory's main claim is that it is more productive to describe a student's cognitive ability in terms of several relatively independent but interacting intelligences than a single 'general' intelligence. With MI theory the question changed from 'how smart is this student?' to 'how is this student smart?' In other words 'what are the relative strengths of this student across all eight intelligences?' However it is important that supporters of the MI model don't fall into the erroneous trap of labelling students by their MI strength in the belief that this will raise their self esteem and motivate them to do well in school. Gardner defines an intelligence as a bio-psychological potential to process particular types of information to solve problems or create products that are valued in at least one culture or community. MI theory identifies the following eight intellectual strengths (Table 2.3).

Each person has an intelligence profile that is a description of their relative strengths and weaknesses across the eight intelligences. According to Moran (2011) what makes the MI approach so powerful is how the different intelligences interact and combine to achieve a purpose. Rich and challenging learning tasks do not isolate one intelligence but rather combine intelligences to achieve a purposeful learning outcome. Take the development of a careers booklet for example. Students are first encouraged to identify their strengths and a career that utilises those strengths (*Intrapersonal intelligence*). The students collaborate in a group of four (*Interpersonal intelligence*) to research, plan and write the booklet (*Verbal-linguistic intelligence*) on four different careers. The booklet contains facts and statistics about different careers (*Logical-mathematical intelligence*) but also strengths and skills checklists to help these students and others assess whether or not they have the capabilities for each career (*Interpersonal and intrapersonal intelligences*). The booklet's graphics and layout engages *visual-spatial intelligence*. Feedback from teacher and other students enhances the participating students' *interpersonal and intrapersonal intelligences*. This exercise also heightens students' sense of purpose by helping them to identify their strengths and target their beliefs about their 'future self'—what career they could aim for, who they could become and ways to become that self. The benefits for students who may face significant barriers to academic success was illustrated in an intervention targeting students in USA from low-income African American and Hispanic 8th graders in an

Table 2.3 Gardner's multiple intelligences	Verbal-linguistic intelligence	Musical intelligence
	Logical-mathematical intelligence	Interpersonal intelligence
	Visual-spatial intelligence	Intrapersonal intelligence
	Bodily-kinaesthetic intelligence	Naturalist intelligence

inner-city school district (Oyserman et al. 2006). The students participated in a 10 session workshop which included describing what kind of adult they would like to be, obstacles they would encounter to becoming that person and how they could overcome those obstacles. Compared to a control group these students earned significantly higher grades in 9th grade, had fewer school absences, were less likely to be reported for disruptive behaviour and were 60 % less likely to repeat 8th grade. Having a sense of purpose in relation to their 'future self' motivated these students to work harder and achieve better grades.

MI theory has been widely adopted in schools across the world since its first publication over thirty years ago (Gardner 1983). The publication *Multiple Intelligences Around the World* (Chen et al. 2009) provides case studies of MI theory applied in education across Asia, Europe, South America and USA. It provides educators with a framework that allows and supports a wider variety of abilities and skills to be expressed and to contribute to the school community than the traditional academic classroom. A differentiated curriculum based on Gardner's multiple intelligences model has the potential to build positive educational communities in which students value and celebrate student differences and for students who struggle with learning to achieve more academic success (Kornhaber et al. 2003; McGrath and Noble 2005a, b; Noble 2004). An evaluation of outcomes in forty-one schools that had been using MI theory for curriculum differentiation for at least three years found significant benefits of the MI approach in terms of improvements in student engagement and learning, student behaviour, and parent participation (Kornhaber et al. 2003). This evaluation found particular benefits for students with learning difficulties who demonstrated greater effort in learning, more motivation and improved learning outcomes when offered different entry points into the curriculum and different ways to demonstrate their understanding of the curriculum.

Gardner advocates the provision of multiple entry points into the curriculum to reach students with different strengths and to raise their level of interest and curiosity in the subject matter. The following table illustrates Gardner's seven entry points with curriculum examples developed by McGrath and Noble (2005a).

Box: Examples of Multiple Entry Points into the Curriculum

Narrative entry point: Telling stories about the topic and people involved e.g. Charles Darwin for evolution; Ernest Shackleton for polar exploration	**Cooperative or social entry point:** e.g: Engaging in cooperative learning groups where each group member's contribution is interdependent on others and everyone collaborates and is accountable
Quantitative entry point: Presenting data connected to the topic such as the twin study correlations for heritability of intelligence or mental illness,	**Aesthetic entry point:** Using powerful visual images or music e.g. analysing visual effects of DVD of Romeo and Juliet, displaying beautiful photos of a

(continued)

(continued)	
or introducing a topic on animals by posing questions about the fastest, heaviest, smallest etc	volcanic eruption or playing music to create a particular mood
Logic entry point: Exploring the logical connections between the key elements e.g. the effects of the sun on water evaporation or photosynthesis	**Hands-on entry point**: Using concrete materials such as blocks to understand mathematical computations, or mixing paint colours to understand the colour wheel
Existential entry point: Addressing the big questions such as the nature of truth or beauty, justice or freedom, life or death	

A curriculum planning tool that helps teachers to plan teaching tasks for different student strengths was developed by McGrath and Noble (1995, 2005a). The curriculum planning tool called the MI/Bloom Matrix (McGrath and Noble 2005a, b) assists teachers to develop tasks based on each of the eight multiple intelligences at each of the six Revised Bloom's levels of thinking (from simple to complex and challenging tasks). The planner helps teachers to provide opportunities for students to make meaningful choices about their learning tasks and products (Noble 2004). The MI/Bloom Matrix is accompanied by a number of MI assessment tools that can be used to assist students to identify their own relative cognitive strengths. The use of the matrix helped all the teachers in two schools identify academic and other strengths in their students and increased the teachers' confidence and skills in diversifying their curriculum tasks to effectively engage their different students in learning (Noble 2004).

Research with teachers in two schools who had used the matrix for over 18 months found that teachers grew in confidence in catering for different student strengths and planning and teaching a diverse range of learning tasks for a differentiated curriculum (Noble 2004). Students were more likely to engage in intellectually challenging activities if they were working in an area of relative strength. Teachers' observations of student engagement and achievements in the diverse learning activities, especially when given an opportunity to work in an area of strength, increased their academic expectations for all students (Noble 2004, 2002). Higher teacher expectations based on curriculum differentiation using multiple intelligences were particularly beneficial for those children from a non-English speaking background or children who struggled with the academic curriculum (Kornhaber et al. 2003; Noble 2004). The following box illustrates the key themes articulated by the teachers in the two research schools who used the MI/Bloom matrix for curriculum differentiation.

Perceived benefits of MI/bloom matrix by teachers
Caters for different student strengths
It (the matrix) helps me to know that I am catering to all the needs in my class because I have a huge range and looking at the activities suggested by the different intelligences (MI) and the levels suggested by Bloom helps me to feel confident that I am catering to those needs
What I like about it (the matrix) is the diversity of tasks. Some children are really extended and go off in directions that you would never even think of. I'm amazed by their creativity
A teacher-friendly planning tool for curriculum differentiation
The matrix helps me to clarify the whole thing in my mind. Just by looking at the matrix you can immediately see the different areas and the different levels and activities and how you are addressing the different intelligences and levels of thinking. It just makes it a clear picture to me; ....If it's clear in my mind in the shape of a matrix, then it's clear in my teaching
A useful tool for planning units of work integrating one or more curriculum areas
The MI/Bloom matrix is fabulous for integrating different curriculum subjects
I'm doing Water as my topic and it's an environment (Social Studies) topic and I'm able to bring in a lot of Language and Science and Technology and Maths such as measuring. Anything like that—it (the matrix) just helps, it gives you ideas to integrate if that's what you want to do
Helps students develop deeper understanding of their ability strengths and the difference between easy and challenging tasks and ways to use and build those strengths
The children got really involved when I started to explain what Bloom was and what Gardner was—I showed them my matrix and where I had placed different activities. They started discussing whether they put this activity there and they were saying things like 'no, that's easier' and then they would turn it around. The kids who really talked it through and developed a better understanding have given me really good work on different tasks. But the other kids who thought it was easy have given me complete rubbish or not what I want. So it's helped some of the kids to talk about what Understand is, what Analyse is, what Space and Vision activities are, Self activities are and so on

2.5.2   Character Strengths

The Values In Action (VIA) model of character strengths developed by Peterson and Seligman (2004) has become popular in positive psychology/positive education. The VIA is based on a review of currently and historically universally valued character traits and defines psychological or character strengths as morally valued traits whose use contributes to fulfilment and happiness (Peterson and Seligman 2004). The VIA shown in the table below incorporates twenty four character strengths organised under six 'virtues' (Table 2.4).

Table 2.4 Peterson and Seligman's character strengths

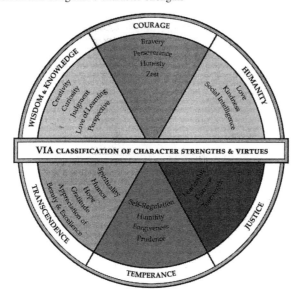

From *Mindfulness and Character Strengths: A Practical Guide to Flourishing* (2014), by Ryan M. Niemiec. Used with permission. All right reserved.
A great colour poster of the strengths can be found at http://www.viacharacter.org/www/Portals/0/poster2.png.

Teachers can help students to identify their character strengths. A useful tool for this purpose is Peterson and Seligman's online VIA (Values in Action) Strengths Questionnaire (www.viacharacter.org). The children's version of the questionnaire is for children from 10 years to 17 years of age. For younger children, Park and Peterson (2006) successfully asked parents of children who were too young to complete the questionnaire to identify their children's strengths. A person's top 3–5 strengths are referred to as their *signature strengths*. A signature strength is defined as a deeply held character trait, that defines one's essence of being. Using our signature strengths are seen to infuse us with energy. They are seen as the core of our identity and thereby help individuals to function at their best and maintain a sense of authenticity (Niemiec 2014).

The use of this framework for fostering wellbeing in school students is relatively new but holds great promise (Quinlan et al. 2014). White and Waters (2014, 2015) presented a case study of a K-12 Australian school that described the potential benefits of a whole school strengths-based approach for enhancing student wellbeing. They outlined how character strengths have been embedded in English literature classes, in the primary curriculum, in sports coaching, in training students for school leadership positions and in counselling students. The authors demonstrated how students from the beginning of their life at school are developing a deep knowledge of how to identify, explore, further develop and apply their character strengths. They argue that the combination of these different initiatives under the umbrella of positive education has contributed to "*a cultural tipping point where the strengths initiatives across the school are fusing to create a strengths-based culture*" (White and Waters 2014, pp. 6–7).

Other examples of the VIA framework used in education include Proctor et al's. (2011) examination of the Strengths gym. Adolescents who participated in exercises in the program that were based around character strengths experienced a significant increase in life satisfaction and positive affect from baseline to post test. The Strath-Haven Positive Psychology program also used the VIA character strengths framework in their Language Arts classes (Seligman et al. 2009). Pre-test to post-test comparisons showed that the students in these classes reported greater enjoyment and engagement in school compared to students in a control group. Teachers also reported that the program improved the students' strengths related to learning such as curiosity, love of learning and creativity and parents and teachers reported improvements in the students' social skills. Quinlan et al. (2014) also describe a six-session classroom-based strengths intervention with 9–12 year old students. Students reported higher levels of positive affect, classroom engagement, autonomy and satisfaction of relatedness needs, class cohesion and strengths use. A useful model for practising character strengths is offered by Niemiec (2014). He provides guidelines on how people can first become 'Aware' of their character strengths, then 'Explore' what it feels like when they engage a strength and finally learn how to 'Apply' the strength in ways that ensures the strength is embedded into life routines. McGrath and Noble (2011a, b) provide examples in the *Bounce Back* program of how teachers can help students, from the first years of schooling, become aware, explore and apply their character and their ability strengths.

2.5.3 Self Respect

Self respect has been defined as a character trait (Ferkany 2007). We define self-respect as an attitude of self-acceptance and approval for one's own character and conduct and consideration for one's own wellbeing. According to Dillon (1997, p. 226)

> individuals who are blessed with a confident respect for themselves have something that is vital to living a satisfying, meaningful, flourishing life, while those condemned to live without it or with damaged or fragile self respect are thereby condemned to live constricted, frustrating lives cut off from possibilities for self-realisation, self-fulfilment and happiness.

As noted in chapter one we suggest that the construct of self respect is a more useful construct for educators and parents than the construct of self esteem. Although the two constructs are similar, the differences between them are crucial (Langer 1999). To esteem anything is to evaluate it positively so self-esteem is an evaluation of one's 'worth' as a person and ranges from low to high. Self-esteem focuses more on successes, what one can do, what one looks like, and/or what one has. Therefore self-esteem fluctuates because it is usually very dependent on feedback from others.

To respect something on the other hand is to accept it. Therefore self respect can be viewed as an attitude of self acceptance. Self respect is not contingent on success because there are always setbacks and failures to deal with; nor is it reliant on comparing ourselves with others because there are always people who are better than us. With self respect we accept ourselves because of who we are and not because of what we can or cannot do.

Young people can be taught to behave in ways that develop and also demonstrate their self-respect. Students with self-respect are more likely to behave in the following ways.

Box: Self Respect

Self-knowledge

They focus more on their strengths than their limitations, work towards self-improvement and don't over-focus on comparing themselves with others. They believe it's OK to be different and OK to be yourself. They consider themselves to be neither inferior nor superior to other people. They continually seek self-knowledge in relation to their ability and character strengths by looking for evidence rather than using 'wishful thinking'.

Self management

They have clear moral values and try to put them into practice. They try not to let themselves down. They try to respond to challenges and difficult times in their life with dignity, courage and resilience. They try to adopt a positive approach to life, focusing on things that go well, expressing gratitude to people who support them and feeling grateful for the good things in their life. They are pleased to receive positive feedback but are not dependent on it nor controlled by it.

They enjoy and feel satisfied with their achievements but avoid being arrogant about them. They balance pride with humility.

Self-protection

They act in ways that protect their physical and psychological safety and their reputation. They believe that they matter and that it is their right to be treated respectfully and fairly and not to be mistreated by others. They are prepared to take appropriate and non-aggressive steps to protect this right. They don't let others put them down and don't put themselves down either. They respect their own body and wellbeing and make an effort to adopt a healthy lifestyle.

Self-kindness

When they feel 'down' they try to be as caring and supportive towards themselves as they would be towards other people they care about. They understand that everyone has self doubts occasionally and they try not to let their self-doubts overwhelm them nor get in the way of achieving their goals. They recognise that they are imperfect but continue to like and accept themselves in spite of difficulties, mistakes or failures; they work hard and feel satisfied with their efforts, even when unsuccessful. They reflect about where they could have managed things differently and try to learn from the experience. They avoid over-criticising themselves and don't give themselves a 'hard time'. They remind themselves about their positive qualities and previous successes.

Self-confidence
They take an optimistic approach when they take on a new or difficult task or challenge. They put in the effort that is required to complete the task and make sure that they have the necessary skills to do it. They use positive self-talk (*e.g. I think I have prepared well enough to be able to do this*) and think realistically but optimistically about any possible risks involved, knowing that they will cope if they don't do as well as they hope.

Self-trust
They trust their own judgment and have faith in themselves; they consider others' viewpoints but are not automatically swayed by them. They try to make sound decisions about what is best for them but also listen to, and incorporate advice and wisdom from people they know they can trust.

Respect and Compassion for Others
They try to treat others with respect and compassion and acknowledge their right to dignity. They accept differences in others and don't see 'differences' as 'defects'. They try to focus more on other people's strengths than their limitations. They don't mistreat or deceive people. They show compassion and support towards others and try to help others in trouble.

2.5.4 Collective Strengths

Moving educational systems and schools from deficit systems to strengths-based systems is a common theme in the literature around school leadership, inclusive schooling, positive psychology, and positive organisational scholarship. A focus on collective strengths and collective responsibility for both student learning and student wellbeing brings together the strengths of the whole educational community in a school including the leadership team, teachers, support staff, administration staff and families. A focus on the collective strengths of everyone in the school contributes to the development of a professional learning community (Hipp and

Huffman 2010). The development of a well-functioning professional learning community has been highlighted as a desirable and perhaps even an essential process within a school for building capacity for improving student achievement (Fullan 2002).

Wenger et al. (2002) described communities of practice as 'groups of people who share a concern, a set of problems or a passion for something they do and who deepen their knowledge and expertise in this area by interacting on a regular basis' (p. 4). The following components of a professional learning community within an educational context have been suggested:

- A collaborative culture with a focus on learning for all and collective enquiry into best practice for teaching and learning (DuFour et al. 2006)
- An action and results orientation and a commitment to continuous improvement (DuFour et al. 2006)
- Supportive and shared leadership (Avenell 2007; Hipp and Huffman 2010)
- Shared values and vision (Bolam et al. 2005)
- Collective learning and the application of that learning (DuFour et al. 2006)
- Shared practice (Mitchell et al. 2001)
- Linkages between school and community (Avenell 2007)
- Supportive conditions that enable ongoing maintenance of the learning community (Fullan 2006).

In practice, a focus on collective strengths often involves processes such as identifying the strengths of individuals and making others aware of these strengths, teachers exchanging feedback about their practice, teachers visiting each other's classrooms and teachers sharing teaching and learning resources.

Technology has facilitated the development and outcomes of professional learning communities, and many educators now extend their professional connections by meeting online with peers to focus, for example, on student wellbeing (see: www.pesa.edu.au). Many learning communities focus on the strengths of people within their school families as well as in the wider community as part of their learning community, embracing and valuing their diverse strengths.

Professional learning communities expect and embrace diversity and value the different strengths of both students and staff. Hoy et al. (2006) research has documented the importance of collective teacher efficacy, also described as 'academic optimism'. Hoy et al's. (2006) research in 96 high schools (Years 9–12) indicated that the teachers' collective academic optimism and their belief that they could improve student learning outcomes enhanced their students' academic achievement and minimised the impact of socio-economic status and other demographic data and the students' previous achievement history. The importance of enhancing teachers' academic optimism and efficacy about their capacity to "make a difference", especially for non-resilient students who are struggling, was also highlighted in a study by Oswald et al. (2003). In this study teachers were more likely to attribute their students' low resilience to personal or family factors rather than factors under their control or a lack of skills that the teacher could teach at school.

Research over the last thirty years or so has clearly demonstrated the effect of teacher expectations on student wellbeing and learning. As Weis and Fine (2003) have observed, low teacher expectations about what students are capable of often reproduces and reinforces social inequalities based on racial, ethnic, social class and gender stereotypes. Seventy four schools in an Australian Priority Action Schools Program (PASP) were identified as schools in communities that had sustained periods of cumulative disadvantage and where community strengths and student wellbeing were not thriving. Many teachers in the PASP program noted that when they took a strengths-based approach and collectively raised their expectations of their students and made their students clearly aware of their raised expectations, these teachers were consistently rewarded by improved student learning performance, keep confidence in their learning increased and their behaviour improved (Groundwater-Smith and Kemmis 2004). One school noted that just supporting students without also intellectually challenging them can lead to 'learned helplessness'. This school demonstrated that a shift to teachers communicating high expectations to their students accompanied by a challenging curriculum was needed to encourage students to reach their 'personal best' levels of performance in both their learning and behaviour.

2.5.5 Using Appreciative Inquiry

Appreciative inquiry (AI) is a collaborative and strengths-based approach to change developed by Cooperrider et al. (2008). It builds on the core principles of the new disciplines of positive psychology and positive education. The approach is built on the assumption that every organisation has a positive core that has contributed to its previous successes as well as its current strengths, potentials and assets. The essence of AI is the art and practice of asking powerful questions that will further strengthen a school's capacity to be a positive learning community.

Appreciative Inquiry is a collaborative, strength-based approach to organisational change and development that energises and motivates individuals to work together to achieve positive outcomes by identifying what's best about the organisation and its people. AI is based on the positive principle that the positive emotions and energy associated with identifying, celebrating, and building on strengths enable people to transform organisations and move them in new directions. In contrast analysing and solving problems can lead to downward spirals of blame and negative energy, whereas discovering and building on collective strengths leads to upward spirals of aspiration, possibility, and the collective efficacy for transformational change (Tschannen-Moran and Tschannen-Moran 2011; Fredrickson 2009). Tschannen-Moran and Tschannen-Moran (2011) provide a comprehensive overview of the use of AI to transform schools and school districts in USA and Europe. The most common version of AI follows 5 stages that are outlined in the following Box.

Box: 5 Stages of appreciative inquiry into student wellbeing in a school

Stage 1: DEFINE (*prior to staff workshop*) The facilitator(s) define the inquiry's key focus. The questions you choose for your AI are crucial to the success of the process, for example:

(i)   how can we enhance student wellbeing within our schools in a cost-effective way?
(ii) how can we improve student achievement at all year levels? or
(iii) how can we improve student engagement in a range of different ways?

Stage 2: DISCOVER (*Individually first; then in small groups; then in the full group*). This 5-step Discovery process is used to discover what can be learnt from the collective past of the participants about 'what has worked well in the past' and what are the 'best features, assets and potentials' of their school that we can build on as we work towards enhancing student wellbeing

1. **Individual Reflections**: Each participant reflects as follows. *'Think back over your experiences at your school (or in other schools); identify a specific situation or experience or a peak time that really stands out for you when you felt energised, satisfied and proud of being associated with the school because it seemed to be 'getting it right' in regards to defined issue. Consider these prompting questions and jot down some notes:*

   - *What was working so well and why? What was happening that contributed?*
   - *What actions were being taken? What structures were in place? What values were being promoted?*
   - *What key people made a difference and how? How did you contribute to the defined issue and what strengths did you use to do so?*

2. **Story-telling In Pairs**: Participants form pairs. One person tells the other person the story of the personal experience/situation/time they have just reflected on. The listener uses prompting questions (see above) and 'tell me more' prompts and takes down some notes. Then they swap over.

3. **Re-telling of Stories in a Group of 4**: Two pairs join up to make groups of four. Each person re-tells their partner's story to the other pair i.e. 4 stories are retold

4. **Group Analysis in the Group of 4**: The 4 people in the group work together to identify the main 'themes' that emerged when their four stories were combined, focusing on:

   - What they have learnt from the past about factors that can 'make a difference' to enhancing student wellbeing
   - What they have identified as the 'best things' (past and present) about their school (e.g. *assets and potential such as people, school*

community, resources, leadership, values etc). These contribute to a school's 'positive core' to be utilised and built on

Each person also has a specific role in this step:

- One person is the group's note-taker and one person will be the spokesperson
- Two people work together to make a mind-map of the themes (*to be placed around the room for viewing by the full group before step 5 begins*)

5. **In the Full Group**: Each group's spokesperson summarises what was 'discovered' about what could make a difference to the defined issue and the best features/assets/potential within their schools that can help to do this. The facilitator creates a list of each group's themes and identifies commonalities.

Stage 3: DREAM (*In the full group*). Participants co-construct a vision of how their school could be if everything they could think of that could contribute to student wellbeing was in place. What would the school and its people look like, act like, think like, feel like?

What would the physical layout and organisation of the school be like? What structures might be in place? How would different teaching and learning processes support this culture? What resources would be available?

Stage 4: DESIGN (*In the full group*). The full group continues to co-construct by identifying the best actions that could be taken to turn the vision into reality. Decisions are made about:

- Two small actions that could be taken immediately that would make a significant difference to student wellbeing
- One 'bold' action that could be taken that has the potential to be a 'game-changer'.
- Who will do what, how and when? How to measure progress and keep it going?
- What ways can everyone in the school 'improvise' informally and make their own contributions to the changes?

Stage 5: DELIVER Make decisions about who will be involved in each of these 'actions' and how and when they will report back. Plan to follow up fairly soon with interim observations/reports.

2.6   PROSPER Pathway 5: Fostering a Sense of PURPOSE

Motivating students to find purpose and meaning in their life is seen as a critical step in enhancing their sense of wellbeing. Purpose is a reliable marker of flourishing (Seligman 2011), thriving (Bundick et al. 2009); psychological wellbeing (Keyes et al. 2002), resilience (Benard 1991; Masten and Reed 2002) and life satisfaction (Mauss et al. 2011; Bronk et al. 2009; Bronk et al. 2010). The two constructs of purpose and meaning share an intention to see one's life as guided by an overarching aim (Steger 2009), and many definitions use the two terms inter-changeably. Finding a sense of purpose in life to shape their sense of identity has long been identified as a primary developmental task for adolescents (Erikson 1968) and an important developmental asset for young people (Benson 2006). In contrast, a life without purpose means that students can drift with no direction (Damon 2008). Moran (2011, p. 123) uses a boat metaphor to explain the difference between being purposeful and purposeless; *"without purpose, a person is like a sailboat, going whichever way the wind blows; with purpose, a young person is like a powerboat, moving forward using a controlled power source toward some marker on the horizon"*. A lack of purpose appears to contribute to poor mental health and is linked to poorer psychological health and higher psychological distress in both young people (e.g. Shek 1993) and adults (e.g. Debats 1998).

Of course it's possible for a young terrorist to have a deep-seated sense of purpose in causing harm to as many people as possible that he perceives do not share his beliefs. He may experience positive emotions, be resilient, be strongly connected to his terrorist gang or organisation, be highly engaged and achieve outcomes deemed as successful by this group and be very satisfied with his life. This example illustrates the importance of Damon's (2008) warning that we should carefully distinguish a noble purpose, which is morally acceptable and admirable, from an ignoble or evil life goal (such as the goal of youth terrorists). Damon defines purpose as *'a stable and generalized intention to accomplish something that is at once meaningful to the self and of consequence to the world beyond the self'* (Damon et al. 2003, p. 121). Therefore purpose indicates engagement in a meaningful activity, perceiving how to extend that activity into the future and having an orientation to have a prosocial impact (Moran 2011). Purpose has three main components: a long-term intention or goal, an action plan and commitment, and a beyond-the-self motivation (Damon 2008).

Research at the Stanford Youth Purpose Project (Malin et al. 2014; Moran 2011) found that only about a quarter of young people aged 12–22 have a sense of purpose in how they can contribute to the big picture and are actually engaged in relevant activities. One in ten understand there is a big picture but they don't know where they fit; and another quarter are oriented to goals like college, jobs, and making money with an intention to benefit primarily themselves. 40 % did not have a clear picture of their strengths, nor a sense of purpose. Not surprisingly non-purposeful students were found more in younger grades, and the purposeful and self-oriented life goal students were more prevalent in 12th grade and college. It would appear that young people who form and sustain a purpose show an exceptional initiative by proactively seeking opportunities and building for themselves a support network to help them achieve their particular purpose (Moran 2011; Malin et al. 2014). According to Moran (2011) it is not so much the particular task or event that is important in fostering a sense of purpose but how the young person perceives and makes use of the initiative. In other words the personal meaning they gain from the experience is more impactful in fostering a sense of purpose than the event itself. The personal meaning the students attribute to the opportunity or challenge facilitates how they perceive the event can contribute positively to others, such as their class, school or local community, now and in the future. Malin et al. (2014) have found that young people with purpose are more likely to talk about seeking out situations to engage their purpose and about how challenges and struggles are opportunities not barriers. For example being teased or bullied or observing bullying might contribute to their drive to make their school a safe and supportive place for everyone.

A sense of purpose also fuels academic tenacity and better academic outcomes. One study that illustrated this encouraged high school students to write in their science lessons every 3 or 4 weeks over a school term a brief essay describing how the content they had studied that week could apply to their lives (Hulleman and Harackiewicz 2009). Students in the intervention group expressed more interest in science at the end of the term and earned higher science grades than students in the control group. Importantly students' grades only improved if the students themselves came up with the reasons why the schoolwork was relevant and not when their teachers simply told them why the material should be relevant to their lives.

So what can schools do to foster a sense of purpose? One example of empowering students to develop a sense of purpose is through their participation in Student Action Teams (Holdsworth et al. 2003). A student action team is a group of students who identify and tackle a school or community issue: they research the issue, make plans and proposals about it, and take action on it (Holdsworth et al. 2003). They demonstrate a sense of purpose by their active engagement in committing time, energy, resources, and knowledge to achieving their goal. To ensure the success of these student-led initiatives Holdsworth et al. (2003) has argued that it is important they are recognized within the 'authorised activities' of a school, and within the 'authorised approaches' of the Education system and not as something that is outside 'proper' school work. Schools that have implemented student action teams indicate a substantial positive change in areas such as knowledge, skills, attitude and connectedness, and students who took part specifically identified their increased level of engagement at school (Holdsworth et al. 2003). Encouraging students to have a deep self knowledge (intrapersonal intelligence) of their character and ability strengths would clearly help them to identify purposeful goals. Moran (2011) argues that without self-understanding young people won't know how to develop, make meaning of or make use of their relative strengths and weaknesses across the eight intelligences. McGrath and Noble (2011a, b Book 3) provide guidelines on how students can work together to use their collective character and ability strengths to help others in their school, local or global community. These guidelines include tools for self reflection on their contributions to their community to enhance their sense of purpose.

Community service (or service learning) is another way schools are facilitating educational experiences that develop student wellbeing and give students a sense of purpose by contributing to the needs and wellbeing of others. Community service has been shown to enhance students' academic skills, transfer of knowledge to 'real world situations', critical thinking skills, as well as a sense of personal and social responsibility and civic engagement, social skills and empathy (Elias et al. 2006; Hanson et al. 2003; Astin et al. 1999; Eyler and Giles 1999). Other school initiatives that can foster a sense of purpose include: encouraging students to participate in peer support programs (e.g. peer mediation, buddy systems, cross-age or same age peer tutoring, mentoring systems); finding ways for students to participate in class-wide or school-wide leadership and decision-making structures such as classroom councils, classroom committees or school-wide Student Representative Committees; arranging for the local community to have access to student products and performances by, for example, organising for students to perform in community centre, displaying their work in a local shopping centre or asking the local library to host a collection of student-made books. Students could also demonstrate their sense of pride in and commitment to their school and local community through the establishment of student-directed 'School Pride 'or 'community pride' Committees' at each year level). All these examples provide real-life, purposeful, problem-solving contributions that illustrate how a student or group of students can and do intentionally and purposefully contribute to their school or local community.

Case Study: Students taking action and gaining a sense of purpose

An academic inquiry unit on '*caring for our environment*' inspired children at one primary school to take action to make a difference in their school and local environment. The children set up their student action team titled the environmental impact team made up of students from kindergarten (5–6 years of age) to year 6 (11–12 years of age). The student action team initiated a number of environmental projects that include (i) a schoolwide 'nude food' campaign where all children are encouraged to bring their lunch to school without plastic wrap; (ii) the installation of 3 rubbish bins in every classroom for (a) recycling, (b) their school worm farm and (c) non-recyclable waste and (iii) a project to raise funds titled '*living gardens*' where the children have made packs of different seeds of herbs and vegetables to sell to their school community. The funds has helped the children set up their own herb and vegetable garden and install chickens in the school grounds as well as buy trees to replant in the local community (Cahill 2012). An interview with Sue Cahill talks about the use of student action teams in their school to reduce school bullying http://www.safeschoolshub.edu.au/safe-schools-toolkit/the-nine-elements/element-7/case-studies/st-charles-ps-element-7/.

A second example at the secondary level was initiated with a group of year 10 students who were disengaged from school and alienated from their neighbourhoods. Appreciative inquiry questions were used to help the students identify their strengths and create purposeful community projects of their choice designed to show how '*we will make a difference in our community*' (Morsilla and Fisher 2007). The projects included a public underage dance party, and the development of children's activities at a refugee cultural festival. These two examples illustrate the key aspects of a Student Action Team; the students are challenged, their participation enables them to make decisions about what's important to them; they learn how to apply their knowledge, skills and attitudes to 'real world' situations; and they gain a real 'authentic' sense of meaning and purpose by contributing to making a difference within their community.

A third example is a *Student Wellbeing Action Group* or SWAG that is a student-initiated and student led group designed to improve student wellbeing across the school. Each year the students in this Government-funded high school held a student wellbeing conference with invited speakers on topics such as cybersafety, or mental health and wellbeing and included the participation of students from 6 other schools. They also initiated a number of school-wide student wellbeing projects such as an anti-bullying campaign. See http://www.safeschoolshub.edu.au/safe-schools-toolkit/the-nine-elements/element-7/case-studies/melbourne-hs-element-7/ for an interview with the SWAG team.

2.7 PROSPER Pathway 6: Enhancing ENGAGEMENT

Engagement can be defined as an observable manifestation of student motivation to learn (e.g. Fredericks et al. 2004; Meyer and Turner 2002). It is most often demonstrated through expression of interest, participation, effort, contribution, enthusiasm and enjoyment. When students don't engage with what is happening at school they can become bored and disaffected or misbehave. In the short term student engagement in learning has been shown to be a reliable predictor of academic outcomes. Over the longer term it is linked to student attendance, academic resilience and school completion (e.g. Jimerson et al. 2003; Klem and Connell 2004). A few studies (e.g. O'Farrell and Morrison 2003) have also suggested that academic engagement may also be protective against the adoption of high-risk student behaviour such as substance abuse. Slade and Trent (2000) established a clear link between student disengagement and pedagogy that was 'boring, repetitive and irrelevant' (p. 221). Fullan (2012) refers to Jenkin's interviews with thousands of teachers that suggested that the level of student engagement drops from 95 % in Kindergarten to 37 % in Grade nine (for a review see Wigfield et al. 2006).

Viewing student engagement from four perspectives can be helpful for educators in planning for curriculum and instruction. Fredricks et al. (2004) talk about behavioural engagement, emotional engagement and cognitive engagement. We add social engagement (McGrath and Noble 2010). When students are highly *behaviourally engaged* they are actively involved and stay absorbed in the learning process. When they are highly *emotionally engaged* in learning in a positive way they are interested, curious, enthusiastic, excited, confident and satisfied with their learning and proud of their learning products. When students are highly *cognitively engaged* they are intellectually challenged and stretched and employing critical and creative thinking. When students are highly *socially engaged* they are positively communicating with their classmates and teacher, cooperating well in a team and using social skills such as turn taking, active listening, and negotiating.

There are qualitative differences in the level or degree of engagement that occurs for each component of engagement (Fredricks et al. 2004). For instance *behavioural engagement* can range from simply doing the work and following rules to actively participating in a student representative council. Similarly emotional engagement can range from simply liking school to deeply valuing their school, social engagement from having one friend to being very popular and well liked. Cognitive engagement can range from simple memorisation to the use of self-regulated learning strategies that promote deep understanding and expertise. These qualitative differences within each dimension indicate that engagement can vary in intensity and duration and be short term and situation specific or long term and stable.

When teachers provided both intellectually challenging and socially supportive environments for all students, their students demonstrate higher levels of engagement, more positive emotions and applied more strategic approaches to their learning (Stipek 2002; Turner et al. 1998). In contrast when teachers focus only on academic content and create a negative social environment, students are more likely to be disengaged and more apprehensive about making mistakes. However if teachers focus only on the social dimensions of a learning task and fail to intellectually challenge students, then they are less likely to be cognitively engaged in learning (Fredricks et al. 2004). Cognitive engagement is enhanced when students have opportunities to actively discuss ideas, debate different points of view and critique each other's work in an emotionally safe learning environment (Guthrie and Wigfield 2000; Meloth and Deering 1994).

2.7.1 Engagement Through Use of Effective Teaching Strategies

The meta-analyses of Hattie (2009) and Marzano et al. (2001), discussed earlier in this section under 'Outcomes' (refer to page 56) also have relevance in terms of enhancing student engagement through the use of effective teaching strategies.

According to Hattie (2009, p. 159) teacher effectiveness is *"less about the content of the curricula and more about the strategies teachers use to implement the curriculum so that students progress upwards through the curricula content"*. Effective evidence-based teaching strategies include cooperative learning, reciprocal teaching and concept mapping (especially when used within a group context (see Box Below).

BOX: Different ways to use concept maps	
Fill in the gaps	Students, working in pairs, are given a half-completed concept map and asked to fill in the missing words and links. Prior preparation by the teacher includes creating a concept map and then identifying which parts to leave out. Each pair will need two copies of the incomplete concept map-one for drafting and one for their final concept map. A list of words that go in the concept map can be provided for some students
Put the jigsaw together	Students work as a pair or group of 3 to put together (e.g. *with blu-tac on a wall or laid out on a desk*) an enlarged concept map 'jigsaw' made by the teacher. The jigsaw components would be text boxes, links and label cards. Each group will need one complete cut-up concept map made from light cardboard
Put this information into a concept map	Students are given a sheet of information and asked to work in a small group to make a concept map to fit that information. Use the DASLER strategy with this version: **D**raft your product **A**gree as a group on why you did it that way **S**hare it with another pair **L**isten to their feedback and give them feedback **E**valuate the feedback **R**evise your product
Start from scratch	Students can be asked to make their own concept map for a specific topic. This can be very challenging!
From: McGrath and Noble (2010)	

Many countries have a crowded educational curriculum. Arguably the most effective teaching strategies are generic strategies that can be used by teachers in any subject at any year level. The content can be any curriculum area whether it is literature, mathematics, history or the sciences. The strategy can combine the social-emotional skills, thinking skills and the technology skills that promote student engagement and student wellbeing. This can be likened to the Russian doll effect where one strategy fits inside another and another and another. The three key ingredients for exceptional teaching that actively engage students in learning fall into three broad categories: *challenge, scaffolding and belonging* (Dweck et al. 2015). Effective teachers and schools *challenge* their students with high performance standards and tasks that promote higher order thinking, provide instructional or cognitive *scaffolding* or motivational *scaffolding* so students can reach the high standard set and cultivate students' sense of *belonging* through the cooperative group structures—a sense of fellowship with their peers and teachers. The topic should be challenging and intrinsically motivating for the students; and the scaffolding and cooperative structure of the teaching strategy are key factors in promoting deep student engagement in learning. The topics that are relevant to real life situations and help promote student voice also help to promote students, sense of purpose in their learning. Highly engaging topics for students are often topics that are values-based controversial or provocative events, issues or 'big ideas', or issues that arise from texts or the media that capture the students' interest (McGrath and Noble 2010) and further their sense of responsibility to their school and their local or global community.

Box: Engagement through use of Higher-order Thinking Tools

The following strategies all combine instructional and cognitive scaffolding that promote critical and/or creative thinking skills, plus scaffolding for cooperative learning and the use of social-emotional skills. (McGrath and Noble 2010). The topics the students research and discuss could readily be issues that contribute to their sense of purpose; for example contributing to a just and peaceful local and global community.

- *Ten Thinking Tracks* is a sequenced cooperative problem-solving/decision making scaffold where students work in groups. Each student in the group takes turns in leading the discussion and recording their group's answers in relation to two or three tracks. The tracks challenge children to think of the bright side, the down side, their feelings, suggest improvements, think ethically and to consider issues of social justice and finally to negotiate a group solution e.g *arranged marriages, microchip for all children under 16 years of age, students to be paid to attend school, no religious clothing or other items to be worn by students to school*
- *Multi-View* encourages perspective taking and empathy. Students consider a problem such as *cyber-bullying, or organ donation from the different perspectives of the people involved.*
- *Under the Microscope* encourages students to explore a controversial issue through different lens that includes their responsibility and the impact of the issue or event on their own lives and on others' lives e.g. *compulsory conscription to army, unemployment benefits.*
- *Cooperative Controversy* provides a scaffold for conflict resolution. Students work in groups of 4 where pair A identifies two arguments in support of a topic-related controversial proposition and pair B identifies two arguments against it. Each pair presents their arguments to the other pair. Then each pair's perspective is reversed and pair A thinks of new

disadvantages and pair B advantages. Finally the group of 4 negotiate the strongest argument for and against. Eg *closing all zoos, compulsory community service for all students*
- In *Socratic circles* half the class becomes the inner circle as discussants and the other half work in the outer circle as observers. The observers have a checklist to provide constructive feedback to the discussants on the quality of their thinking and their use of social-emotional skills. The two groups then swap roles and responsibilities e.g. *can school bullying be eradicated from all schools, why are so many people homeless?*

From: McGrath and Noble (2010).

Engagement through technology. The digital world of the 21st century is a highly engaging one for students, providing opportunities for 'any time, any place' learning 24 h per day, 7 days a week. Dewey's famous quotation' *if we teach today as we were taught yesterday, we rob our children of tomorrow* (Dewey 1944, p. 167) *has* more relevance now than ever before. Educators need to keep pace with technology to keep students actively engaged in learning. Helping children learn how to use technology are essential skills in the 21st century. Engagement can be enhanced through learning activities that promote online communication with children in other classes, schools and countries, social networking and the use of gaming principles. Students' use of ICT also increases their capacity to take responsibility for their own learning and to be creative and innovative in the way they learn, in defining problems, in problem solving and decision-making and in the multi-media products they produce. Through technology students can now connect and collaborate with children in other parts of the world. For example primary school aged children can now work collaboratively with others in different countries to compare the different seasons across countries or study different ways of celebrating birthdays or other key events. Secondary aged students can collaborate to engage in a discussion of world issues by videoconferencing with students from the countries in which they are occurring. Such experiences can enhance children's capabilities to be more creative problem solvers, self-directed learners, better communicators and life long learners. They can also be challenged to develop a greater capacity for empathy and social justice as they become more aware of different local and global perspectives.

Technology also offers a cost-effective way of helping students in impoverished or remote communities access education without the requirements for the physical infrastructure that has limited learning opportunities in the past. Providing internet facilities in local libraries, sponsoring the reconditioning of old computers so they can be sold more cheaply within needy communities, offering free training courses for young people and adults hosted by schools, and teaching about new technologies all encourage greater involvement with online education. The potential benefits from such initiatives are especially valuable for children and young people in remote communities who have access to ICT but not access to high quality schooling.

Although many low and middle-income countries have limited access to personal computers, the majority of the world's population now have access to a mobile cellular signal and around 40 % have access to mobile broadband (ITU 2013). The extraordinary worldwide uptake of mobile subscriptions grew from less than 1 billion in 2000 to 6 billion in 2011 of which nearly 5 billion were in low and middle income countries (World Bank 2012; Layard and Hagell 2015). The UN estimates that more people have access to mobile phones than a toilet (6 billion compared with 4.5 billion respectively) (UN News Center 2013). Hence the potential for the development of mobile telephone apps is vast—30 billion were downloaded in 2011 and the number is rising (Layard and Hagell 2015). Layard and Hagell are strong advocates for the development and distribution of mobile apps designed to enhance the mental health and wellbeing of children. Examples of two Australian organisations developing such apps to enhance youth mental health and wellbeing are Reachout (www.reachout.com) and the Young and Well Foundation. The potential of such apps is that billions of children and their teachers and parents could access these apps anywhere in the world. The role of an adult such as a teacher or parent is still pivotal to ensure that children understand and have opportunities to apply the app's key messages, especially for young children in the early and primary years. Two programs, one in India and one in Kenya illustrate the benefits of technology for engaging children in education in developing countries. Both programs use media, including television, radio, and comics to teach literacy skills and to connect and educate young people through the power of storytelling.

Case Study

Planet Read-India

India ranks 147th out of 177 countries for literacy based on UNESCO data. Hundreds of millions in India are either illiterate, or 'neo-literates'—possessing only rudimentary literacy skills despite having attended several years of primary school. Recognizing that literacy skills have to be constantly reinforced, *Planet Read* appropriated the method of 'Same Language Subtitling' (SLS)—the practice of subtitling television programs, films or video clips in the same language as the audio track—and applied it to the wildly popular Bollywood music videos aired weekly on television throughout the country.

With hundreds of millions of viewers keen to learn the words to their favorite songs, *Planet Read's* program has a huge reach. When exposed to 30 min of SLS per week, the functional literacy rate among students who had at least five years of Hindi schooling grew from 25 to 56 %. The organization estimates that its weekly broadcasts reach an audience of approximately 200 million neo-literates nationwide. http://theglobaljournal.net/article/view/508/.

Well Told Story-Kenya

Well Told Story engages Kenyan youth (more than half of Kenyans are under 18, and nearly three quarters are under 30) via a multi-media approach, that includes a monthly comic, a Facebook page, downloads for mobile phones, and a daily syndicated radio show. The multi-media approach engages different segments of their young audience, and helps motivate young people to more engaged forms of media participation and real world action. The radio show and comic reaches out to Kenyan youth with practical ideas on how they can improve their lives. The subjects that have been the focal point have ranged from seed soaking, to helping street children, to national cohesion. http://www.welltoldstory.co.ke.

2.7.2   Engagement and 'Flow'

'Flow' is a term coined by Csikszentmihalyi (2002) that defines a high level of engagement with an activity. People are more likely to be fully engaged and experience 'flow' when involved in an activity that utilises their strength(s) and has a degree of challenge that requires a reasonably high level of skill (Csikszentmihalyi et al. 1993). Being in a state of 'flow' increases students' satisfaction with the completion of a task, whether it be a complex puzzle, a research activity, or the creation of a product or performance. 'Flow' also has the potential to provide some respite from worries and problems that a student may be experiencing. Tasks that engage student strengths in the service of others have the potential to create flow and at the same time provide a sense of meaning and purpose.

Students experience flow when they are so immersed in an intrinsically rewarding activity that hours pass like minutes, their mind is totally focused and they are completely absorbed in the activity. A student who is fully engaged with a learning task finds it enjoyable, may practise or study it a lot and is more likely to persist with it despite challenges (Nakamura and Csikszentmihalyi 2005). Athletes often refer to this state as 'being in the zone' and it occurs when they encounter a sporting challenge that they know that they have the skills to meet. If the challenge of a task exceeds a student's level of skill, he/she may become anxious and disengage from the task. If their skills exceed the challenge of the task, then they are likely to be bored and this can also lead to disengagement. This may occur, for example, when highly able students are in class in which the teacher has a 'one-size-fits-all' approach rather than an approach based on curriculum differentiation. Activities in which a student can use his/her strengths are especially likely to produce 'flow'.

2.8   PROSPER Pathway 7: Teaching RESILIENCE

All students face adversity at one time or other. Typically these difficult times are related to family or friendship changes or losses, poor academic performance and setbacks and disappointments when things don't go their way (e.g. not being selected to be part of a team or cast of a play or missing out on an award). Some students also have more serious adversity to deal with such as ongoing poverty and disadvantage, abuse or serious illness. Resilience has been defined as '*the ability to persist, cope adaptively and bounce back after encountering change, challenges, setback, disappointments, difficult situations or adversity and to return to a reasonable level of wellbeing. It is also the capacity to respond adaptively to difficult circumstances and still thrive*' (McGrath and Noble 2011a). Skills for being resilient are essential for both academic and personal success in school and in life. The resilient skills that can be taught to students are: optimistic thinking skills, helpful thinking skills, adaptive distancing skills, using humour and seeking assistance when needed (McGrath and Noble 2011a).

- *Optimistic thinking skills*: MacLeod and Moore (2000) have concluded that an optimistic way of interpreting and adjusting to negative life events is an essential component of resilience. Hope and an optimistic explanatory style are two components to optimistic thinking for school-based resilience programs. *Hope is* having a disposition to *expect* things to work out, and to be proactive and persist when faced with setbacks or adversity (Carver and Scheier 1999). *An optimistic explanatory style* is believing that bad situations are temporary, acknowledging that bad situations are usually not all your fault, and believing that bad situations are specific, and don't affect everything else or necessarily flow over into all aspects of your life (Gillham and Reivich 2004; Seligman et al. 1995). These skills have been outlined in greater detail under 'Positivity'
- *Helpful thinking* is rational thinking based on reality, not on how an individual would like things to be. Such thinking helps a student feel more emotionally in control and hence be more able to solve problems. It's underpinned by Cognitive Behaviour Therapy model (CBT) (Beck 1979) based on the understanding that how you think affects how you feel which in turn influences how you behave.
- *Adaptive distancing* includes being able to detach from individuals whose influence is negative (Werner and Smith 1992) and finding ways to emotionally distance oneself from distressing and unalterable situations instead of constantly immersing oneself in a negative situation and continually thinking about it.

The Bounce Back program (McGrath and Noble 2011a) illustrates how the teaching of resilience can be embedded in the school curriculum. It is a whole school kindergarten to middle school program that integrates the use of CBT principles for teaching resilience in a curriculum unit called *People Bouncing Back* with 8 other units. The other units are *Looking on the Bright Side* that teaches optimistic thinking: *Courage; Core Values; Emotions; Relationships; Humour; No Bullying* and *Success* (strengths and goal setting linked to purpose). The implementation of the program in 16 primary schools in Scotland enhanced students' personal resilience skills, social skills and class connectedness, as well as teacher wellbeing and contributed to the development of a more positive and school culture with higher levels of peer acceptance (Axford et al. 2011). Similarly it's implementation in 18 bushfire-affected schools after the devastating 2009 Australian bushfires with great loss of life and property demonstrated an increase in students' capacity to behave more confidently, resiliently and pro-socially (McGrath and Noble 2011b). There is also an adapted version of Bounce Back! for colleges.

Dweck and her colleagues (Dweck 2006; Yeager and Dweck 2012; Blackwell et al. 2007) have shown that low resilience impacts negatively on students' academic and social outcomes. Low academic resilience is linked to students developing a fixed mindset where they perceive their intelligence is unchangeable. In contrast, high academic resilience is linked to a growth mindset. A growth versus fixed mindset in regard to intelligence shapes students' *goals* (whether they are eager to learn and grow or care more about looking smart or at least not looking dumb); their *beliefs about effort* (whether effort is perceived as the key to success and growth or a signal that they lack natural talent), their *attributions* for their setback (whether a setback means they need to work harder and alter their strategies or whether it means they are 'dumb') and their *learning strategies* in face of setbacks (whether they work harder or give up, cheat and/or become defensive). Blackwell et al. (2007) showed that these variables explained why students with a growth mindset were more resilient and achieved higher grades. Dweck's model of a 'growth mindset' is also addressed under 'Outcomes'.

Similarly students' 'mindsets' can influence their social resilience. Yeager and Dweck (2012) found that students who were bullied or excluded by their peers and who had a 'fixed mindset' about their personality saw the situation as unchangeable, concluding that they must be unlikable and those who were being mean to them must be nasty people. These students not only reacted more negatively in the short term to this social adversity but also showed high levels of stress, worsening health and lower grades over the school year. However other students who were also bullied or excluded but who had 'a growth mindset' in regard to their personality and the social behaviour of the other students, were significantly less likely to endorse aggressive vengeful responses and reported feeling fewer negative emotions such as shame or hatred. Although attempts to teach students to adopt a 'resilience mindset' have been successful, Yeager and Dweck (2012) have warned that such training needs to be customised for different student populations. For example Blackwell et al. (2007) improved high school students' growth mindset by teaching them that greater effort in learning could strengthen their brains. However

Yeager and Dweck (2012) found that college students frequently put forth great effort but used very poor strategies and do not ask for help. Teaching these students to focus on *effort + strategy + help from others* significantly improved their results and course completion.

2.8.1 PROSPER: Pulling It All Together

PROSPER is a useful organising framework for assisting schools and teachers to be self-reflective and act as change agents by addressing the components in the framework to enhance students' capacity to flourish and thrive. The box below suggests some key questions that need to be asked

Box: Teacher Reflection on School Practices that assist students to PROSPER

PROSPER pathways	Reflection on practice
Positivity Supporting students to develop a positive mindset and experience positive emotions	What actions can I take to ensure that students: • Feel safe and have a sense of belonging? • Feel curious and interested about what they are learning? • Feel satisfied with their learning experiences? • Experience a sense of fun, pleasure and amusement? • Learn skills for mindfulness? • Learn to feel and express gratitude and appreciation? • Develop skills in positive tracking, positive reframing, optimistic thinking and hopefulness
Relationships Supporting students to develop the social skills and pro-social values that underpin positive relationships and building positive relationships within the school	What actions can I take to: • Build positive relationships with my students? • Develop positive relationships with my colleagues? • Teach pro-social values and social-emotional skills to guide how we all interact with each other? • Use more cooperative learning structures so that students learn, play and work successfully together in a variety of contexts?
Outcomes Provision of an optimal learning environment to enhance students' outcomes and accomplishment	What actions can I take to: • Help students to develop 'grit' and a 'growth mindset' with a focus on effort, willpower and persistence? • Use more evidence-informed approaches that have been shown to be effective teaching strategies • Include more formative assessment in my teaching • Give students opportunities to co-develop assessment criteria and provide more helpful feedback about their learning
Strengths Taking a strengths-based approach with students,	What actions can I take to: • Provide a differentiated curriculum for students with different ability strengths

(continued)

(continued)

PROSPER pathways	Reflection on practice
teachers and the whole school community	• Embed a focus on students' character strengths in the curriculum, and through different school practices • Help students to identify, explore and apply their character and ability strengths • Acknowledge and build on the strengths of my colleagues
Purpose Supporting students to develop a sense of purpose and meaning	What actions can I take to: • Help students formulate a purposeful 'beyond-the-self' goal and support them to achieve their plan commitment • Encourage student autonomy, initiative and student voice • Help students self-reflect on the big picture purpose or future purpose of their activities
Engagement Providing opportunities for high levels of student engagement	What actions can I take to: • Increase my students' engagement with the curriculum • Ensure my students are challenged in their area of strength(s) • Use more evidence-informed approaches in my teaching to maximise student engagement
Resilience Supporting students to develop the skills and attitudes that underpin resilient behaviour	What actions can I take to: • Help students to develop a 'resilience mindset' • Teach students the skills and attitudes that will enable them to be more resilient in both their academic and personal lives

References

Astin, A. W., Sax, L. J., & Avalos, J. (1999). Long-term effects of volunteerism during the undergraduate years. *Review of Higher Education, 22*(2), 187–202.

Avenell, K. (2007). Common themes on learning communities. *The Australian Educational Leader, 29*(1), 46–47.

Axford, S., Schepens, R., & Blyth, K. (2011). Did introducing the Bounce Back Programme have an impact on resilience, connectedness and wellbeing of children and teachers in 16 primary schools in Perth and Kinross, Scotland? *Educational Psychology, 12*(1), 2–5.

Banas, J. A., Dunbar, N., Rodriguez, D., & Liu, S. (2011). A review of humor in education settings: Four decades of research. *Communication Education, 60*(1), 115–144.

Barclay, J. R., & Doll, B. (2001). Early prospective studies of the high school dropout. *School Psychology Quarterly, 16*(4), 357–369.

Battistich, V. (2001). *Effects of an elementary school intervention on students' 'Connectedness' to school and social adjustment during middle school.* Paper presented at the annual meeting of the American Educational Research Association, Seattle, April.

Battistich, V., Schaps, E., Watson, M., Solomon, D., & Lewis, C. (2001). Effects of the child develop-ment project on students' drug use and other problem behaviours. *Journal of Primary Prevention, 21*, 75–99.

Battistich, V., Schaps, E., & Wilson, N. (2004). Effects of an elementary school intervention on students' "connectedness" to school and social adjustment during middle school. *Journal of primary prevention., 24*(3), 243–262.

Battistich, V., Solomon, D., Kim, D., Watson, M., & Schaps, E. (1995). Schools as communities, poverty levels of student populations, and students' attitudes, motives and performance: A multilevel analysis. *American Educational Research Journal, 32*, 627–658.

Baumeister, R. F., & Leary, M. R. (1995). The need to belong: Desire for interpersonal attachments as a fundamental human motivation. *Psychological Bulletin, 117*, 497–529.

Baumeister, R. F., & Tierney, J. (2011). *Willpower: Why success is the secret of success.* UK: Penguin.

Beck, A. T. (1979). *Cognitive therapy and the emotional disorders.* New York: Penguin.

Becker, B. E., & Luthar, S. S. (2002). Social-emotional factors affecting achievement outcomes among disadvantaged students: Closing the achievement gap. *Educational Psychologist, 37*(4), 197–214.

Benard, B. (1991). *Fostering resiliency in kids: Protective factors in the family, school and community.* San Francisco, CA: Western Regional Center for Drug Free Schools and Communities. Far West Laboratory.

Benard, B. (2004). *Resiliency: What we have learned.* San Francisco: WestEd.

Bennett, M. P., & Lengacher, C. (2008). Humor and laughter may influence health: III. *Laughter and Health Outcomes Evid Based Complement Alternat Med., 5*(1), 37–40.

Benninga, J. S., Berkowitz, M. W., Kuehn, P., & Smith, K. (2003). The relationships of character educa- tion and academic achievement in elementary schools. *Journal of Research in Character Education, 1*(1), 17–30.

Benson, P. L. (2006). *All kids are our kids: What communities must do to raise caring and responsible children and adolescents* (2nd ed.). San Francisco, CA: Jossey Bass.

Bergin, C., & Bergin, D. (2009). Attachment in the classroom. *Educational Psychological Review., 21*, 141–153.

Berk, L. S. (2001). Modulation of neuroimmune parameters during the eustress of humor-associated mirthful laughter. *Alternative Therapies in Health and Medicine, 7*(2), 6–13.

Bishop, S. R., Lau, M., Shapiro, S. L., Carlson, L., Anderson, N. D., Carmody, J., & Devins, G. (2004). Mindfulness: A proposed operational definition. *Clinical Psychology: Science and Practice, 11*, 230–241.

Bizumic, B., Reynolds, K. J., & Turner, J. C. (2009). The role of the group in individual functioning: School identification and the psychological well-being of staff and students. *Applied Psychology. An International Review, 58*(1), 171–192.

Blackorby, J., & Wagner, M. (1996). Longitudinal post-school outcomes of youth with disabilities: Findings from the National Longitudinal Transition Study. *Exceptional Children, 62*(5), 399–414.

Blackwell, L. S., Trzesniewski, K. H., & Dweck, C. S. (2007). Implicit theories of intelligence predict achievement across an adolescent transition: A longitudinal study and an intervention. *Child Development, 78*(1), 246–263.

Blum, R. W., & Libbey, H. P. (2004a). School connectedness—strengthening health and education outcomes for teenagers. *Journal of School Health, 74*, 231–235.

Blum, R. W., & Libbey, H. P. (2004b). Wingspread declaration on school connections. *Journal of School Health, 74*, 233–234.

Boivin, M., Hymel, S., & Bukowski, W. M. (1995). The roles of social withdrawal, peer rejection, and victimisation by peers in predicting loneliness and depressed mood in childhood. *Development and Psychopathology, 7*, 765–785.

Bolam, R., McMahon, A., Stoll, L., Thomas, S., & Wallace, M. (2005). *Creating and sustaining effective professional learning communities.* London, UK: DfES.

Bollmer, J. M., Milich, R., Harris, M. J., & Maras, M. A. (2005). A friend in need: The role of friendship quality as a protective factor in peer victimization and bullying. *Journal of Interpersonal Violence., 20*(6), 701–712.

Bond, L., Butler, H., Thomas, L., Carlin, J., Glover, S., Bowes, G., & Patton, G. C. (2007). Social and school connectedness in early secondary school as predictors of late teenage substance use, mental health, and academic outcomes. *Journal of Adolescent Health, 40*(357), 9–18.

Bond, L., Carlin, J. B., Thomas, L., Rubin, K., & Patton, G. C. (2001). 'Does bullying cause emotional problems? A prospective study of young teenagers'. *British Medical Journal, 323*, 480–484.

Booth-Butterfield, M., Booth-Butterfield, S., & Wanzer, M. (2007). Funny students cope better: Patterns of humor enactment and coping effectiveness. *Communication Quarterly, 55*, 299–315.

Bosworth, K., Espelage, D. L., & Simon, T. R. (1999). Factors associated with bullying behavior in middle school students. *Journal of Early Adolescence, 19*(3), 341–362.

Bower, J. M., van Kraayenoord, C., & Carroll, A. (2014). Building social connectedness in schools: Australian teachers' perspectives. *International Journal of Educational Research, 70*, 101–109.

Bradshaw, C., Koth, C., Bevans, K., Ialongo, N., & Leaf, P. (2008). The impact of school-wide positive behavioral interventions and supports (PBIS) on the organizational health of elementary schools. *School Psychology Quarterly, 23*(4), 462–473.

Bradshaw, C., Koth, C., Thornton, L., & Leaf, P. (2009). Altering school climate through school-wide positive behavioral interventions and supports: Findings from a group-randomized effectiveness trial. *Prevention Science, 10*, 100–115.

Brigman, G., & Webb, L. (2007). Student success skills: Impacting achievement through large and small group work. *Journal of Group Dynamics: Theory, Practice and Research, 11*, 283–292.

Bronk, K. C., Finch, W. H., & Talib, T. (2010). The prevalence of a purpose in life among high ability adolescents. *High Ability Studies, 21*(2), 133–145.

Bronk, K. C., Hill, P. L., Lapsley, D. K., Talib, T. L., & Finch, H. (2009). Purpose, hope, and life satisfaction in three age groups. *Journal of Positive Psychology, 4*(6), 500–510.

Bryant, F. B., & Veroff, J. (2007). *Savoring: A new model of positive experience.* Mahwah, NJ: Lawrence Erlbaum.

Bundick, M. J., Yeager, D. Y., King, P., & Damon, W. (2009). Thriving across the life span. In W. F. Overton & R. M. Lerner (Eds.), *Handbook of lifespan human development.* New York, NY: Wiley.

Cahill, S. (2012). Interview with Sue Cahill at St Charles Borromeo School, Melbourne, Australia. http://www.safeschoolshub.edu.au/safe-schools-toolkit/the-nine-elements/element-7/case-studies/st-charles-ps-element-7/

Caprara, G. V., Barbaranelli, C., Pastorelli, C., Bandura, A., & Zimbardo, P. G. (2000). Prosocial foundations of children's academic achievement. *Psychological Science, 11*(4), 302–306.

Carr, D. (2006). Professional and personal values and virtues in teaching. *Oxford Review of Education, 32*(2), 171–183.

Carver, C. S., & Scheier, M. F. (1999). Stress, coping, and self-regulatory processes. In L. A. Pervin & O. P. John (Eds.), *Handbook of personality* (2nd ed., pp. 553–575). New York: Guilford.

Catalano, R. F., Kosterman, R., Hawkins, J. D., et al. (1996). Modelling the etiology of adolescent substance use: A test of the social development model. *Journal of Drug Issues, 26*, 429–455.

Cemalcilar, Z. (2010). Schools as socialization contexts: Understanding the impact of school climate factors on students' sense of school belonging. *Applied Psychology: An International Review, 59*(2), 243–272.

Charney, R. (2002). *Teaching children to care: Classroom management for ethical and academic growth, K-8.* Greenfield, MA: Northeast Foundation for Children.

Chen, J., Moran, S., & Gardner, H. (Eds.). (2009). *Multiple intelligences around the world.* San Francisco, CA: Jossey-Bass.

Clifton, D. O., & Harter, J. K. (2003). Investing in strengths. In A. K. Cameron, B. J. Dutton, & C. R. Quinn (Eds.), *Positive organizational scholarship* (pp. 111–121). San Francisco: Berrett-Koehler Publishers Inc.

Cohen, J., Pickeral, T., & Levine, P. (2010). The foundation for democracy: Promoting social, emotional, ethical, cognitive skills and dispositions in K-12 school. *Interamerican Journal of Education for Democracy., 3*(1), 74–94.

Colom, G., Alcover, C., Sanchez-Curto, C., & Zarate-Osuna, J. (2011). Study of the effect of positive humour as a variable that reduces stress. Relationship of humour with personality and performance variables. *Psychology in Spain, 15*(1), 9–21.

Cooperrider, D. L., Whitney, D., & Stavros, J. M. (2008). *AI handbook for leaders of change* (2nd ed.). Brunswick, OH: Crown.

Cornelius White, J. (2007). Learner-centered teacher–student relationships are effective: A meta-analysis. *Review of Educational Research, 77*(1), 113–143.

Cowie, H., & Olafsson, R. (2000). The role of peer support in helping the victims of bullying in a school with high levels of aggression. *School Psychology International, 21*, 79–95.

Criss, M. M., Pettit, G. S., Bates, J. E., Dodge, K. A., & Lapp, A. L. (2002). Family adversity, positive peer relationships, and children's externalizing behaviour: A longitudinal perspective on risk and resilience. *Child Development, 73*, 1220–1237.

Croninger, R. G., & Lee, V. E. (2001). Social capital and dropping out of high schools: Benefits to at-risk students of teachers' support and guidance. *Teachers College Record., 103*(4), 548–581.

Cross, D., Hall, M., Hamilton, G., Pintabona, Y., & Erceg, E. (2004). Australia: The friendly schools project. In P. K. Smith, D. Pepler, & K. Rigby (Eds.), *Bullying in schools: How successful can interventions be?* (pp. 187–210). Cambridge: Cambridge University Press.

Cross, D., Shaw, T., Hearn, L., Epstein, M., Monks, H., & Lester, L., et al. (2009). *Australian Covert Bullying Prevalence Study* (ACBPS), Child Health Promotion Research Centre, Edith Cowan University, Perth. Retrieved June 4th, 2009, from www.deewr.gov.au/Schooling/NationalSafeSchools/Pages/research.aspx

Csikszentmihalyi, M. (2002). *Flow: The classic work on how to achieve happiness.* London: Rider.

Csikszentmihalyi, M., Rathunde, K., & Whalen, S. (1993). *Talented teenagers.* Cambridge, UK: Cambridge University Press.

Damon, W. (2008). *The path to purpose. How young people find their calling in life.* NY: Simon Schuster.

Damon, W., Menon, J., & Bronk, K. C. (2003). The development of purpose during adolescence. *Applied Developmental Science, 7*(3), 119–128.

Davis, H. (2003). Conceptualizing the role and influence of student–teacher relationships on children's social and cognitive development. *Educational Psychologist, 38*(4), 207–234.

Debats, D. L. (1998). Measurement of personal meaning: The psychometric properties of the life regard index. In P. T. P. Wong & P. S. Fry (Eds.), *The human quest for mean- ing: A handbook of psychological research and clinical applications* (pp. 237–259). Mahwah, NJ: Lawrence Earlbaum.

Deci, E. L., & Ryan, R. M. (1985). *Intrinsic motivation and self-determination in human behaviour.* NY: Plenum.

Deci, E. L., & Ryan, R. M. (2000). The" what" and" why" of goal pursuits: Human needs and the self-determination of behavior. *Psychological Inquiry, 11*(3), 227–239.

Dewey, J. (1944). *Democracy and education.* New York: Macmillan Company.

Dillon, R. S. (1997). Self-respect: Moral. *Emotional and Political. Ethics, 107*(2), 226–249.

Doll, B., & Hess, R. S. (2001). Through a new lens: Contemporary psychological perspectives on school completion and dropping out. *School Psychology Quarterly, 16*(4), 351–356.

Donohue, K. M., Perry, K. E., & Weinstein, R. S. (2003). Teachers' classroom practices and children's rejection by their peers. *Journal of Applied Developmental Psychology, 24*(1), 91–118.

Dorman, J. P., & Ferguson, J. M. (2004). Associations between students' perceptions of mathematics classroom environment and self-handicapping in Australian and Canadian high schools. *McGill Journal of Education, 39*(1), 69–86.

Duckworth, A., Grant, H., Loew, B., Oettingen, G., & Gollwitzer, P. M. (2011). Self-regulation strategies improve self-discipline in adolescents: benefits of mental contrasting and implementation intentions. *Educational Psychology, 31*(1), 17–26.

Duckworth, A., & Seligman, M. E. P. (2005). Self-discipline outdoes IQ in predicting academic performance of adolescents. *Psychological Science, 16*(12), 939–944.

DuFour, R., Eakey, R., & Many, T. (2006). *Learning by Doing A handbook for professional learning communities at work.* USA: Solution Tree.

Dweck, C. S. (2006). *Mindset. The New Psychology of Success.* New York: Random House.

Dweck, C. S., Walton, G. M., & Cohen, G. L. (2015). Academic Tenacity. *Mindsets and skills that promote long-term learning*. Bill & Melinda Gates Foundation. https://web.stanford.edu/~gwalton/home/Welcome_files/DweckWaltonCohen_2014.pdf

Elias, M., & Zins, J. (2003). Bullying, other forms of peer harrassment, and victimization in the schools: Issues for school psychology research and practice. In M. Elias & J. Zins (Eds.), *Bullying, peer harrassment, and victimization in the schools: The next generation of prevention*. Binghamton, New York: Haworth Press.

Elias, J. E., Zins, P. A., Graczyk, R. P., & Weissberg, R. (2003). Implementation, sustainability, and scaling up of social-emotional and academic innovations in public schools. *School Psychology Review, 32*, 303–319.

Elias, M. J., Zins, J. E., Weissberg, R. P., Frey, K. S., Greenberg, M. T., Haynes, N., et al. (2006). *Promoting social and emotional learning: Guidelines for educators*. VA ASCD: Alexandria.

Emmons, R. A. (2007). *Thanks! How the new science of gratitude can make you happier*. New York: Houghton, Mifflin Co.

Emmons, R. A., & Shelton, C. M. (2002). Gratitude and the science of positive psychology. In C. R. Synder & S. J. Lopez (Eds.), *Handbook of positive psychology* (pp. 459–471). New York: Oxford University Press.

Endresen, I. M., & Olweus, D. (2001). 'Self-reported empathy in Norwegian adolescents: Sex differences, age trends, and relationship to bullying'. In A. C. Bohart & D. J.Stipek (Eds.), *Constructive and destructive behavior: Implications for family, school and society* (pp. 147–165). Washington, DC: American Psychological Association.

Engels, R. C., Finkenauer, C., Meeus, W., & Dekovic, M. (2001). Parental attachment and adolescents' emotional adjustment: The associations with social skills and relational competence. *Journal of Counselling Psychology, 48*(4), 428–439.

Erikson, E. H. (1968). *Identity, youth and crisis*. New York: WW Norton.

Espelage, D. C., Mebare, S., & Adam, R. (2004). Empathy and the bully-victim continuum. In D. L. Espelage & S. M. Swearer (Eds.), *Bullying in American schools: A social ecological perspective on prevention and intervention* (pp. 37–61). Laurence Erlbaum Associates: Mahwah NJ.

Espelage, D. L., & Swearer, S. M. (2003). Research on school bullying and victimization: What have we learned and where do we go from here? *School Psychology Review, 32*(2), 365–383.

Eyler, J. & Giles, D. (1999). *Where's the learning in service-learning*. San Francisco: Jossey-Bass Publisher.

Farrington, D. P., & Ttofi, M. M. (2009). School-based programs to reduce bullying and victimization. *Campbell Systematic Reviews, 5*(6).

Felson, R. B., Liska, A. E., South, S. J., & McNulty, T. L. (1994). The subculture of violence and delinquency: Individual vs. school context affects. *Social Forces, 73*(1), 155–173.

Ferkany, M. A. (2007). The nature and importance of self-respect. *Dissertation Abstracts International Section A: Humanities and Social Sciences. 68*(4-A), *1485*.

Flannery, D., Vazsonyi, A. T., Liau, A. K., Guo, S., Powell, K. E., Atha, H., et al. (2003). Initial behaviour outcomes for the peace builders universal school-based violence prevention program. *Developmental Psychology, 39*(2), 292–308.

Flashpohler, P. D., Elfstrom, J. L., & Vanderzee, K. L. (2009). Stand by me: The effects of peer and teacher support in mitigating the impact of bullying on quality of life. *Psychology in the Schools, 46*, 636–649.

Fredricks, J. A., Blumenfeld, P. C., & Paris, A. H. (2004). School engagement: Potential of the concept, state of the evidence. *Review of Educational Research, 74*, 59–109.

Fredrickson, B. (2009). *Positivity*. New York: Crown Publishing Group.

Fredrickson, B. (2013). Positive emotions broaden and build. *Advances in Experimental Social Psychology, 47*, 1–53.

Fredrickson, B. L., Cohn, M. A., Coffey, K. A., Pek, J., & Finkel, S. M. (2008). Open hearts build lives: Positive emotions induced through loving-kindness mediation, build consequential personal resources. *Journal of Personal and Social Psychology, 95*(5), 1045–1062.

Fredrickson, B. L., & Losada, M. F. (2005). Positive affect and the complex dynamics of human flourishing. *American Psychologist, 60*(7), 678–686.

Fredrickson, B., & Tugade, M. (2004). Resilient individuals use positive emotions to bounce back from negative emotional experiences. *Journal of Personality and Social Psychology, 86*(2), 320–333.

Froh, J. J., & Bono, G. (2011). Gratitude in youth: A review of gratitude interventions and some ideas for applications. *NASP Communique, 39* (5). Retrieved March 3, 2015, from www.nasponline.org/publications/cq/mocq395GratitudeinYouth.aspx

Froh, J. J., Bono, G., & Emmons, R. A. (2010). Being grateful is beyond good manners: Gratitude and motivation to contribute to society among early adolescents. *Motivation and Emotion, 34*, 144–157.

Froh, J. J., Emmons, R. A., Card, N. A., Bono, G., & Wilson, J. A. (2011). Gratitude and the reduced costs of materialism in adolescents. *Journal of Happiness Studies, 12*, 289–302.

Froh, J. J., Sefick, W. J., & Emmons, R. (2008). Counting blessings in early adolescents, An experimental study of gratitude and subjective wellbeing. *Journal of School Psychology, 46*, 213–233.

Fullan, M. (2002). Beyond instructional leadership: The change leader. *Educational Leadership, 59*(8), 16–21.

Fullan, M. (2006). The future of educational change: System thinkers in action. *Journal of Educational Change, 7*(3), 113–122.

Fullan, M. (2012). *Stratosphere, integrating technology*. Pearson: Pedagogy and Change Knowledge.

Furrer, C., & Skinner, E. (2003). Sense of relatedness as a factor in children's academic engagement and performance. *Journal of Educational Psychology, 95*(1), 148–162.

Garaigardobil, M., Magento, C., & Etxeberria, J. (1996). Effects of a co-operative game program on socio-affective relations and group cooperation capacity. *European Journal of Psychological Assessment., 12*, 141–152.

Gardner, H. (1983). *Frames of mind*. New York: Basic Books.

Gardner, H. (2006). *Multiple intelligences: New horizons*. New York: Basic Books.

Garmezy, N. (1991). Resilience in children's adaptation to negative life events and stressed environments. *Pediatric Annals, 20*(9), 459–463.

Gillham, J., & Reivich, K. (2004). Cultivating optimism in childhood and adolescence. *The Annals of the American Academy of Political and Social Science, 59*, 146–163.

Gini, G., Albiero, P., Benelli, B., & Altoe, G. (2007). Does empathy predict adolescents' bullying and defending behavior? *Aggressive Behavior, 33*, 467–476.

Ginsburg-Block, M. D., Rohrbeck, C. A., Fantuzzo, J. W. (2006). A meta-analytic review of social, self-concept, and behavioral outcomes of peer-assisted learning. *Journal of Educational Psychology, 98*(4), 732–749.

Goodenow, C. (1993). The Psychological sense of school membership among adolescents: Scale development and educational correlates. *Psychology in the Schools, 30*(1), 79–90.

Govindji, R., & Linley, P. (2007). Strengths use, self-concordance and well-being: Implications for strengths coaching and coaching psychologists. *International Coaching Psychology Review, 2*, 143–153.

Greco, L., & Morris, T. L. (2005). Factors influencing the link between social anxiety and peer acceptance: Contributions of social skills and close friendships during middle childhood. *Behaviour Therapy, 36*(2), 197–205.

Greenberg, M., Weissberg, R., O'Brien, M., Zins, J., Fredericks, L., Resnik, H., & Elias, M. (2003). Enhancing school-based prevention and youth development through coordinated social, emotional, and academic learning. *American Psychologist, 58*, 466–474.

Gregory, A., Cornell, D., Fan, X., Sheras, P., Shih, T-H., & Huang, F. (2010). Authoritative school discipline: High school practices associated with lower bullying and victimization. *Journal of Educational Psychology, 102*(2), 483–496.

Gresham, F. M. (1986). Conceptual issues in the assessment of social competence in children. In P. S. Strain, M. J. Guralnick, & H. M. Walker (Eds.), *Children's social behaviour* (pp. 143–180). New York: Academic Press.

Groundwater-Smith, S., & Kemmis, S. (2004). *Knowing makes the difference: Learnings from the NSW priority action schools program (PASP).* NSW Department of Education and Training. Accessed June 4th, 2008.

Gruwell, E., & Freedom Writers. (1999). The freedom writer's diary: How a teacher and 150 teens used writing to change themselves and the world around them. New York: Broadway Books.

Gurland, S. T., & Grolnick, W. S. (2003). Children's expectancies and perceptions of adults: Effects on rapport. *Child Development, 74,* 1212–1224.

Guthrie, J. T., & Wigfield, A. (2000). Engagement and motivation in reading. In. M. L. Kamil, P. B. Mosenthal, P. D. Pearson, & R. Barr (Eds.), *Hand-book of reading research* (3rd. ed., pp. 403–422). New York: Longman.

Hamre, B. K., & Pianta, R. C. (2001). Early teacher-child relationships and the trajectory of children's school outcomes through eight grade. *Child Development, 72*(2), 625–638.

Hanson, T., Austin, G. & Lee-Bayha, J. (2003). *Student health risks, resilience and academic performance in California.* Safe and Healthy Kids Program Office, California: West Ed.

Hartup, W. W., & Stevens, N. (1997). Friendships and adaptation in the life course. *Psychological Bulletin, 121,* 355–370.

Hattie, J. (2009). *Visible learning: A synthesis of over 800 meta-analyses relating to achievement.* London: Routledge.

Hatzichristou, C., & Hopf, D. (1996). A multi-perspective comparison of peer sociometric status groups in childhood and adolescence. *Child Development, 67,* 1085–1102.

Hill, T. (1989). Neglected and rejected children: Promoting social competence in early childhood settings. *Australian Journal of Early Childhood, 14*(1), 11–16.

Hipp, K. A., & Huffman, J. B. (Eds.). (2010). *Demystifying professional communities: School leadership at it's best.* NY: Roman & Littlefield.

Hodges, E. V. E., Boivin, M., Vitaro, F., & Bukowski, W. M. (1999). The power of friendship: Protection against an escalating cycle of peer victimization. *Developmental Psychology, 35*(1), 94–101. doi:10.1037/0012-1649.35.1.94.

Holdsworth, R., Cahill, S., & Smith, G. (2003). *Student action teams, An evaluation of implementation and impact.* Parkville: Faculty of Education, University Melbourne.

Horner, R. H., Sugai, G., Smolkowski, K., Eber, L., Nakasato, J., Todd, A. W., & Esperanza, J. (2009). A randomized, wait-list controlled effectiveness trial assessing school-wide positive behavior support in elementary schools. *Journal of Positive Behavior, 11*(3), 133–144.

Howells, K. (2012). *Gratitude in education. A radical view.* Rotterdam: Sense Publishers.

Howes, C., & Ritchie, S. (1999). Attachment organizations in children with difficult life circumstances. *Development and Psychopathology, 11,* 251–268.

Hoy, W. K., Tarter, C. J., & Woolfolk-Hoy, A. W. (2006). Academic optimism of schools: A force for student achievement. *American Educational Research Journal., 43*(3), 425–446.

Hughes, J. N., Cavell, T. A., & Wilson, V. (2001). Further evidence of the developmental significance of the teacher–student relationship. *Journal of School Psychology, 39,* 289–302.

Hulleman, C. S., & Harackiewicz, J. M. (2009). Promoting interest and performance in high school science classes. *Science, 326,* 1410–1412.

Implementing the National Framework for Values Education in Australian Schools. (2006). Final report. Retrieved March 3rd, 2015, from http://www.valueseducation.edu.au/verve/_resources/VEGPS1_FINAL_REPORT_081106.pdf

International Telecommunications Union (ITU). (2013). *Measuring the information society.* Available from http://www.itu.int/en/ITU-D/Statistics/Documents/publications/mis2013/MIS2013_without_Annex_4.pdf

Janson, G. R., Carney, J. V., Hazler, R. J., & Oh, I. (2009). Bystanders reactions to witnessing repetitive abuse experiences. *Journal of Counseling and Development, 87,* 319–326.

Jimerson, S. R., Campos, E., & Greif, J. L. (2003). Toward an understanding of definitions and measures of school engagement and related terms. *California School Psychologist, 8,* 7–27.

Johnson, D., & Johnson, R. (2009). An educational psychology success story: Social interdependence theory and cooperative learning. *Educational Researcher, 38*, 365. http://er. aera.net

Jolliffe, D., & Farrington, D. P. (2006). Examining the relationship between low empathy and bullying. *Aggressive Behavior, 32*, 540–550.

Jones, M. G., & Gerig, T. M. (1994). Silent sixth-grade students: Characteristics, achievement, and teacher expectations. *The Elementary School Journal, 95*(2), 169–182.

Joyce, H. D., & Early, T. J. (2014). The impact of school connectedness and teacher support on depressive symptoms in adolescents: A multilevel analysis. *Children and Youth Services Review, 39*, 101–107.

Juvonen, J. (2006). Sense of belonging, social relationships, and school functioning. In A. P. Alexander & P. H. Winne (Eds.), *Handbook of educational psychology* (2nd ed., pp. 655–674). NJ: Lawrence Erlbaum Associates.

Keddie, A., & Churchill, R. (2003). Power, control and authority: Issues at the centre of boys' relationships with their teachers. *Queensland Journal of Teacher Education, 19*(1), 13–27.

Keyes, C. L. M., Shmotkin, D., & Ryff, C. D. (2002). Optimizing well-being: The empirical encounter of two traditions. *Journal of Personality and Social Psychology, 82*, 1007–1022.

Klem, A. M., & Connell, J. P. (2004). Relationships matter: Linking teacher support to student engagement and achievement. *Journal of School Health, 74*(7), 262–273.

Konishi, C., Hymel, S., Zumbo, B. D., & Li, Z. (2010). Do school bullying and student–teacher relations matter for academic achievement?: A multilevel analysis. *Canadian Journal of School Psychology, 25*, 19–39.

Kornhaber, M., Fierros, E., & Veenema, S. (2003). *Multiple Intelligences: Best ideas from research and practice*. Boston: Allyn & Bacon.

Krause, K., Bochner, S., & Duchesne, S. (2006). *Educational psychology for learning and teaching* (2nd ed.). Southbank, Victoria: Nelson Australia Pty Ltd.

La Greca, A., & Harrison, H. (2005). Adolescent peer relations, friendships, and romantic relationships: Do they predict social anxiety and depression? *Journal of Clinical Child & Adolescent Psychology, 34*(1), 49–61.

Ladd, G. W. (1990). Having friends, keeping friends, making friends, and being liked by peers in the classroom: Predictors of children's early school adjustment? *Child Development, 61*, 1081–1100.

Ladd, G. (2003). Probing the adaptive significance of children's behavior and relationships in the school context: A child by environment perspective. *Advances in Child Development and Behavior, 31*, 43–104.

Ladd, G. W., & Burgess, K. B. (2001). Do relational risks and protective factors moderate the linkages between childhood aggression and early psychological and school adjustment? *Child Development, 72*, 1579–1601.

Ladd, G., Kochenderfer, B., & Coleman, C. (1997). Classroom peer acceptance, friendship, and victimization: Distinct relational systems that contribute uniquely to children's school adjustment? *Child Development, 68*, 1181–1197.

Langer, E. (1999). Self-esteem vs. Self-respect. The Power Lies in the Difference. *Psychology Today*, November/December.

Lavery, L. (2008). Self-regulated learning for academic success: An evaluation of instructional techniques. PhD thesis, University of Auckland, New Zealand.

Layard, R., & Hagell, A. (2015). Healthy young minds: Transforming the mental health of children. In J. H. Helliwell, R. Layard & J. Sachs (Eds.), *World Happiness Report 2015*. New York: Sustainable Development Solutions Network. www.unsdsn.org/happiness

Linley, A., & Harrington, S. (2006). Playing to your strengths. *The Psychologist, 19*, 86–89.

Lopez, S. J., Rose, S., Robinson, C., Marques, S., & Pais Reibero, J. (2009). Measuring and promoting hope in schoolchildren. In R. Gilman, E. S. Huebner & Furlong, M (Eds.), *Promoting wellness in children and youth: Handbook of positive psychology in the schools*. Mahwah, New Jersey: Lawrence Erlbaum.

Lovat, T., & Clement, N. (2008). Quality teaching and values education: Coalescing for effective learning. *Journal of Moral Education, 37*(1), 1–16.

Lovat, T., & Toomey, R. (2007). *Values education and quality teaching: The Double Helix effect.* Sydney: David Barlow.

Lyubomirsky, S., Diener, E., & King, C. (2005). The benefits of frequent positive affect: Does happiness lead to success? *Psychological Bulletin, 131*(6), 803–855.

Macleod, A. K., & Moore, R. (2000). Positive thinking revisited: Positive cognitions, well- being and mental health. *Clinical Psychology & Psychotherapy, 7*, 1–10.

Malin, H., Reilly, T. S., Quinn, B., & Moran, S. (2014). Adolescent purpose development: Exploring empathy, discovering roles, shifting priorities, and creating pathways. *Journal of Research on Adolescence, 24*, 186–199. doi:10.1111/jora.12051.

Marcus, R. F., & Sanders-Reio, J. (2001). The influence of attachment on school completion. *School Psychology Quarterly, 16*, 427–444.

Marks, H. M. (2000). Student engagement in instructional activity: Patterns in the elementary, middle, and high school years. *American Educational Research Journal, 37*, 153–184.

Martin, R. A. (2006). *The psychology of humor.* NY: Academic Press.

Martin, A., Marsh, H., McInerney, D., Green, J., Dowson, M. (2007). Getting along with teachers and parents: The yields of good relationships for students' achievement motivation and self-esteem. *Australian Journal of Guidance and Counselling, 17*(2), 109–125.

Marzano, R. J. (2003). *What works in schools: Translating research into action.* Alexandria, VA: Association for Supervision and Curriculum Development.

Marzano, R. J., Marzano, J. S., & Pickering, D. (2003). *Classroom management that works: Research-based strategies for every teacher.* Alexandria, VA: Association for Supervision and Curriculum Development.

Marzano, R. J., Pickering, D. J., & Pollock, J. E. (2001). *Classroom instruction that works: Research-based strategies for increasing student achievement.* Alexandria, VA: Association for Supervision and Curriculum Development.

Masten, A. S., & Obradović, J. (2008). Disaster preparation and recovery: Lessons from research on resilience in human development. *Ecology and Society, 13*(1), 9.

Masten, A. S., & Reed, M. G. (2002). Resilience in development. In C. R. Snyder & S. J. Lopez (Eds.), *The handbook of positive psychology* (pp. 74–88). New York: Oxford University Press.

Mauss, I. B., Shallcross, A. J., Troy, A. S., John, O. P., Ferrer, E., Wilhelm, F. H., et al. (2011). Don't hide your happiness! Positive emotion dissociation, social connectedness, and psychological functioning. *Journal of Personality and Social Psychology, 100*(4), 738–748.

McDougall, P., Hymel, S., Vaillancourt, T., & Mercer, L. (2001). The consequences of childhood rejection. In M. R. Leary (Ed.), *Interpersonal rejection* (pp. 213–247). New York, NY: Oxford University Press.

McGrath, H. L. (2007). *Schools without Bullying: Can it Really Happen?* Paper presented at ACEL/ASCD Educational Leadership Conference, Sydney.

McGrath, H., & Francey, S. (1991). *Friendly kids, friendly classrooms.* Melbourne: Pearson Education.

McGrath, H. & Noble, T. (1995). *Seven ways At once.* Melbourne: Pearson Education.

McGrath, H., & Noble, T. (2005a). *Eight ways at once. Book One: Multiple Intelligences + Bloom's Revised Taxonomy = 200 differentiated classroom strategies.* Sydney: Pearson Education.

McGrath, H., & Noble, T. (2005b). *Eight ways at once. Book Two: Units of Work Based Multiple Intelligences + Bloom's Revised Taxonomy* Sydney: Pearson Education.

McGrath, H., & Noble, T. (2010). *HITS and HOTS. Teaching + Thinking + Social Skills.* Pearson Education: Melbourne.

McGrath, H., & Noble, T. (2011a). *Bounce Back! A wellbeing & resilience program. Lower primary K-2; Middle primary: Yrs 3–4; Upper primary/Junior secondary: Yrs 5-8.* Melbourne: Pearson Education.

McGrath, H. & Noble, T. (2011b). Report of the evaluation of the impact of training teachers in bushfire-affected schools to use the bounce back classroom resiliency program in their classrooms. NSW: Victorian Department of Education and Early Childhood.

McGrath, H., Stanley, M., & Craig, S. (2005). *Review of anti-bullying policy and practice.* Victoria: Department of Education and Training.

McInerney, D. M., & McInerney, V. (2006). *Educational psychology: Constructing learning* (4th ed.). Frenchs Forrest, NSW: Pearson Education Australia.

Meiklejohn, J., Phillips, C., Freedman, M. L., Griffin, M. L., Biegel, G., Roach, A., & Saltzman, A. (2012). Integrating mindfulness training into K-12 education: Fostering the resilience of teachers and students. *Mindfulness, 3*(4), 291–307.

Meloth, M. S., & Deering, P. D. (1994). Task talk and task awareness under different learning conditions. *American Educational Research Journal, 31*(1), 138–165.

Menesini, E., Codecasa, E., Benelli, B., & Cowie, H. (2003). Enhancing children's responsibility to take action against bullying: Evaluation of a befriending intervention in Italian middle schools. *Aggressive Behavior, 29*(1), 1–14.

Meyer, D. K., & Turner, J. C. (2002). Discovering emotion in classroom motivation research. *Educational Psychologist, 37,* 107–114.

Miltich, A. P., Hunt, M. H., & Meyers, J. (2004). Dropout and violence needs assessment: A follow-up study. *The California School Psychologist, 9,* 131–140.

Mishima, K. (2003). Bullying amongst close friends in elementary school. *Japanese Journal of Social Psychology, 19,* 41–50.

Mishna, F., Weiner, J., & Pepler, D. (2008). Some of my best friends: Experiences of bullying within friendships. *School Psychology International, 29,* 549–573.

Mitchell, J., Wood, S., & Young, S. (2001). Communities of practice reshaping professional practice and improving organisational productivity in the vocational education and training (VET) sector. Australian National Training Authority.

Moran, S. (2011). Measuring multiple intelligences and moral sensitivities in education. *Moral Development and Citizenship Education., 5,* 121–133.

Morrison, M. K. (2008). *Using humor to maximize learning: The links between positive emotions and education.* Maryland, U.S.A.: Rowman & Littlefield Education.

Morsilla, J., & Fisher, A. (2007). Appreciative inquiry with youth to create meaningful community projects. *The Australian Community Psychologist, 19*(1), 47–61.

Mueller, C. M., & Dweck, C. S. (1998). Intelligence praise can undermine motivation and performance. *Journal of Personality and Social Psychology, 75,* 33–52.

Nadel, J., & Muir, D. (2005). *Emotional development: Recent research advances.* Oxford: Oxford University Press.

Nakamura, J., & Csikszentmihalyi, M. (2005). The concept of flow. In C. R. Snyder & S. J. Lopez (Eds.), *Handbook of positive psychology* (pp. 89–105). New York: Oxford University Press.

Neuliep, J. W. (1991). An examination of the content of high school teachers' humor in the classroom and the development of an inductively derived taxonomy of classroom humor. *Communication Education, 40,* 343–355.

Newman, R. S. (1991). Goals and self-regulated learning: What motivates children to seek academic help? In M. L. Maehr & P. R. Pintrich (Eds.), *Advances in motivation and achievement: Goals and self-regulatory processes* (pp. 151–184). New York: Academic Press.

Niemiec, R. M. (2014). *Mindfulness and character strengths.* Boston, MA: Hogrefe Publishing.

Noble, T. (2004). Integrating the revised bloom's taxonomy with multiple intelligences: A planning tool for curriculum differentiation. *Teachers College Record., 106*(1), 193–211.

Noddings, N. (1992). *The challenge to care in schools: An alternative approach to education.* New York: Teachers College Press.

NSSF: National Safe Schools Framework. (2011a). *Ministerial council for education, early childhood development and youth affairs.* Retrieved March 1, 2015, from http://www.safeschoolshub.edu.au/documents/nationalsafeschoolsframework.pdf

NSSF: National Safe Schools Framework. (2011b). http://www.deewr.gov.au/schooling/nationalsafeschools/Pages/overview.aspx

O'Farrell, S. L., & Morrison, G. M. (2003). A factor analysis exploring school bonding and related constructs among upper elementary students. *California School Psychologist, 8*, 53–72.

O'Malley, M., Katz, K., Renshaw, T., & Furlong, M. (2012). Gauging the system: Trends in school climate measurement and intervention. In S. Jimerson, A. Nickerson, M. Mayer, & M. Furlong (Eds.), *The handbook of school violence and school safety: International research and practice* (2nd ed., pp. 317–329). New York: Routledge.

Oettingen, G. (2014). *Rethinking positive thinking. Inside the new science of motivation.* NY: Penguin.

Ollendick, T. H., Weist, M. D., Borden, M. C., & Greene, R. W. (1992). Sociometric status and academic, behavioral, and psychological adjustment: A five-year longitudinal study. *Journal of Consulting and Clinical Psychology, 60*, 80–87.

Osterman, K. F. (2000). Students' need for belonging in the school community. *Review of Educational Research, 70*, 323–367.

Oswald, M., Johnson, B., & Howard, S. (2003). Quantifying and evaluating resilience promoting factors: Teachers' beliefs and perceived roles. *Research in Education, 70*, 50–64.

Oyserman, D., Bybee, D., & Terry, K. (2006). Possible selves and academic outcomes: How and when possible selves impel action. *Journal of Personality and Social Psychology, 91*, 188–204.

Park, N., & Peterson, C. (2006). Character strengths and happiness among young children: Content Analysis of parental descriptions. *Journal of Happiness Studies, 7*, 323–341.

Peterson, C. (2013). *Pursuing the good life.* NY: Oxford University Press.

Peterson, C., & Seligman, M. E. P. (2004). *Character strengths and virtues: A handbook and classification.* Oxford: Oxford University Press.

Phillips, L. (2008). *Provoking critical awareness and intersubjectivity through 'Transformational storytelling'.* Paper presented at AARE conference.

Pianta, R. (1999). *Enhancing relationships between children and teachers* (1st ed.). Washington, DC: American Psychological Association.

Pianta, R. C., Belsky, J., Vandergrift, N., Houts, R. M., & Morrison, F. J. (2008). Classroom effects on children's achievement trajectories in elementary school. *American Educational Research Journal, 45*(2), 365–397.

Pianta, R., & Walsh, D. (1996). *High-risk children in schools: Constructing and sustaining relationships.* New York: Routledge.

Proctor, C., Tsukayama, E., Wood, A. M., Maltby, J., Eades, J. F., & Linley, P. A. (2011). Strengths gym: The impact of a character strengths-based intervention on the life satisfaction and well-being of adolescents. *The Journal of Positive Psychology, 6*, 377–388.

Quinlan, D. M., Swain, N., Cameron, C., & Vella-Brodrick, D. A. (2014). How 'other people matter' in a classroom-based strengths intervention: Exploring interpersonal strategies and classroom outcomes. *The Journal of Positive Psychology,*. doi:10.1080/17439760.2014.920407.

Raskauskas, J., Gregory, J., Harvey, S., Rifshana, F., & Evans, I. (2010). Bullying among primary school children in New Zealand: Relationships with prosocial behaviour and classroom climate. *Educational Research, 52*(1), 1–13.

Resnick, M. D., Bearman, P. S., & Blum, R. W. (1997). Protecting adolescents from harm: Findings from the National Longitudinal Study on Adolescent Health. *JAMA, 278*, 823–832.

Rhodes, J. E., Grossman, J. B., & Resch, N. L. (2000). Agents of change: Pathways through which mentoring relationships influence adolescents' academic adjustment. *Child Development, 71*(6), 1662–1671.

Rimm-Kaufman, S. (2011). *Improving students' relationships with teachers to provide essential supports for learning.* American Psychological Association. Retrieved October 6, 2014, from http://www.apa.org/education/k12/relationships.aspx

Roorda, D. L., Koomen, H. M. Y., Spilt, J. L., & Oort, F. J. (2011). The influence of affective teacher–student relationships on students' school engagement and achievement: A meta-analytic approach. *Review of Educational Research, 8*, 493–529.

Roseth, C. J., Johnson, D. W., & Johnson, R. T. (2008). Promoting early adolescents' achievement and peer relationships: The effects of cooperative, competitive and individualistic goal structures. *Psychological Bulletin, 134*(2), 223–246.

Rowe, K. (2004). In good hands? The importance of teacher quality. *Educare News, 149,* 4–14.

Rudasill, K. M., Rimm-Kaufman, S. E., Justice, L. M., & Pence, K. (2006). Temperament and language skills as predictors of teacher-child relationship quality in preschool. *Early Education and Development, 17*(2), 271–291.

Ryan, R. M., & Deci, E. L. (2000). Self-determination theory and the facilitation of intrinsic motivation, social development, and well-being. *American Psychologist, 55,* 68–78.

Schonert-Reichl, K. A. (1999). Moral reasoning during early adolescence: Links with peer acceptance, friendship, and social behaviors. *Journal of Early Adolescence, 19,* 249–279.

Schwartz, S. H. (2011). Values: Cultural and individual. Fundamental question in cross—cultural psychology. Cambridge University Press, Cambridge.

Schwartz, D., Dodge, K. A., Pettit, G. S., & Bates, J. E. (2011). Friendship as a moderating factor in the pathway between early harsh home environment and later victimisation in the peer group. *Developmental Psychology, 36,* 646–662.

Seligman, M. E. P. (1991). *Learned optimism.* New York: Knopf.

Seligman, M. E. P. (1995). The effectiveness of psychotherapy: The consumer reports study. *American Psychologist, 50,* 965–974.

Seligman, M. E. (2011). *Flourish: A visionary new understanding of happiness and wellbeing.* NY: Simon and Schuster.

Seligman, M. E. P., Ernst, R. M., Gillham, J., Reivich, K., & Linkins, M. (2009). Positive education: Positive psychology and classroom interventions. *Oxford Review of Education, 35* (3), 293–311.

Seligman, M. E. P., Reivich, K., Jaycox, L., & Gillham, J. (1995). *The optimistic child.* New York: Houghton Mifflin.

Shek, D. T. (1993). The Chinese purpose-in-life test and psychological well-being in Chinese college students. *International Forum for Logotherapy, 16,* 35–42.

Simmel, G. (1996). Faithfulness and gratitude. In A. Komter (Ed.), *The gift: An interdisciplinary perspective.* Amsterdam: Amsterdam University Press.

Slade, M., Trent, F. (2000). What the boys are saying: An examination of the views of boys about declining rates of achievement and retention. *International Education Journal, 1*(2).

Snyder, C. R., & Lopez, S. J. (2007). *Positive psychology: The scientific and practical explorations of human strengths.* Thousand Oaks, CA, US: Sage Publications.

Stanley, M., & McGrath, H. (2006). Buddy systems: Peer support in action. In H. McGrath & T. Noble (Eds.), *Bullying solutions; Evidence-based approaches for Australian schools.* Sydney: Pearson Education.

Steger, M. F. (2009). Meaning in life. In S. J. Lopez (Ed.), *Handbook of positive psychology* (2nd ed.). Oxford, UK: Oxford University Press.

Stipek, D. (2002). Good instruction is motivating. In A. Wigfield & J. Eccles (Eds.), *Development of achievement motivation.* California: Academic Press.

Stipek, D. (2006). Relationships matter. *Educational Leadership, 64*(1), 46–49.

Sugai, G., Horner, R., & Lewis, T. (2009). *School-wide positive behaviour support implementers' blueprint and self-assessment.* Eugene, OR: OSEP TA-Center on Positive Behavioral Interventions and Supports.

Swearer, S. M., & Cary, P. T. (2007). Perceptions and attitudes toward bullying in middle school youth: A developmental examination across the bullying continuum. In J. E. Zins, M. J. Elias, & C. A. Maher (Eds.), *Bullying, victimization, and peer harassment* (pp. 67–83). New York: Haworth Press.

Swearer, S. M., & Doll, B. (2001). Bullying in schools: An ecological framework. *Journal of Emotional Abuse, 2*(2/3), 7–23.

Thapa, A., Cohen, J., Higgins-D'Alessandro, A., & Guffey, S. (2012). School climate research summary. NY: National School Climate Center. www.schoolclimate.org

Thoma, S. J., & Ladewig, B. H. (1993). *Moral judgment development and adjustment in late adolescence*. Atlanta, GA: Paper presented to the American Educational Research Association.

Trent, F. (2001). *Aliens in the classroom or: The classroom as an alien place?* Paper presented as the Association of Independent Schools, NSW Sex, Drugs & Rock N Roll Conference, August http://www.studentnet.edu.au/aispd/resources/Faith_Trent.pdf

Turner, J. C., Meyer, D. K., Cox, K. E., DiCintio, M., & Thomas, C.T. (1998). Creating contexts for involvement in mathematics. *Journal of Educational Psychology, 90*, 730–745.

Tschannen-Moran, M., & Tschannen-Moran, B. (2011). Taking a strengths-based focus improves school climate. *Journal of School Leadership, 21*(3), 422–448. http://www.schooltransformation.com/wp-content/uploads/2012/06/Strengths-Improve-Climate.pdf

UN News Center. [Online press release]. (2013). *Deputy UN Chief calls for urgent action to tackle global sanitation crisis*. March 21, 2013, Available at www.un.org/apps/news/story.asp?NewsiD=44452#.VF9erzQgt8E

Weare, K. (2000). *Promoting mental, emotional and social health. A whole school approach*. London: Routledge.

Weis, L., & Fine, M. (2003). Extraordinary conversations in public schools. In G. Dimitriadis & D. Carlson (Eds.), *Promises to keep: Cultural studies, democratic education, and public life* (pp. 95–123). New York: RoutledgeFalmer.

Weissberg, R., Caplan, M., & Harwood, R. (1991). Promoting competent young people in competence-enhancing environments: A systems-based perspective on primary prevention. *Journal of Consulting and Clinical Psychology, 59*(6), 830–841.

Wenger, E., McDermott, R., & Synder, R. W. (2002). *Cultivating communities of practice: A guide to managing knowledge*. Boston: Harvard Business School Press.

Wentzel, K. R., & Asher, S. R. (1995). The academic lives of neglected, rejected, popular, and controversial children. *Child Development, 66*, 754–763.

Wentzel, K. R., & Caldwell, K. (1997). Friendships, peer acceptance, and group membership: Relations to academic achievement in middle school. *Child Development, 68*, 1198–1209.

Wentzel, K. R., & Watkins, D. E. (2002). Peer relationships and collaborative learning as contexts for academic enablers. *School Psychology Review, 31*(3), 336.

Werner, E. E. (2002). Looking for trouble in paradise: Some lessons learned from the Kauai Longitudinal Study. In E. Phelps, F. F. Furstenberg, A. Colby (Eds.), *Looking at lives: American longitudinal studies of the 20th century* (pp. 297–314). New York: Russell Sage Foundation.

Werner, E., & Smith, R. (1992). *Overcoming the odds: High risk children from birth to adulthood*. New York: Adams, Bannister and Cox.

White, M., & Waters, L. E. (2014). A case study of 'The Good School:' Examples of the use of Peterson's strengths-based approach with students. *The Journal of Positive Psychology,* doi:10.1080/17439760.2014.920408.

White, M., & Waters, L. E. (2015). Strengths-based approaches in the classroom and staffroom. In M. A. White & A. S. Murray (Eds.), *Evidence-based approaches in positive education*. Positive Education, doi:10.1007/978-94-017-9667-5_6

Wigfield, A., Eccles, J. S., Schiefele, U., Roeser, R., & Davis-Kean, P. (2006). Development of achievement motivation. In W. Damon (Series Ed.) & N. Eisenberg (Vol. Ed.), *Handbook of child psychology: Vol. 3. Social, emotional, and personality development* (6th ed., pp. 933–1002). New York: Wiley.

Wood, A. M., Linley, A. P., Maltby, J., Kashdan, T. B., & Hurling, R. (2011). Using personal and psychological strengths leads to increases in wellbeing over time: A longitudinal study and the development of the strengths use questionnaire. *Personality and Individual Differences, 50*, 15–19.

World Bank. (2012). *Information and communications for development 2012: Maximizing mobile*. Available from http://bit.ly/1pAfMiW

Yeager, D. S., & Dweck, C. S. (2012). Mindsets that promote resilience: When students believe that personal characterics can be developed. *Educational Psychologist, 47*(4), 302–314.

Yeager, J., Fisher, S., & Shearon, D. (2011). *Smart strengths: Building character, resilience and relationships in youth.* New York: Kravis Publishing.

Yovetich, N., Dale, A., & Hudak, M. (1990). Benefits of humor in reduction of threat-induced anxiety. *Psychological Reports, 66,* 51–58.

Zins, J. E., Weissberg, R. P., Wang, M. C., & Walberg, H. J. (Eds.). (2004). *Building academic success on social and emotional learning: What does the research say?* New York: Teachers College Press.

Chapter 3
Policy Development for Student Wellbeing

Abstract This chapter reviews the common objections and potential risks attached to a student wellbeing policy and the importance of taking an evidence-informed approach. An overview of the benefits of a student wellbeing policy is then presented, followed by guidelines/actions for developing a student wellbeing policy at the school, system, national and international levels.

Keywords School policy · Student wellbeing · International policy

3.1 Introduction

The wellbeing of students should be the explicit goal of every school. It is hard to think of a more deserving cause than the wellbeing of children worldwide (Layard and Hagell 2015). Such a goal requires a whole school approach to student wellbeing. This means that everyone in the school community, students, teachers, support staff, parents and carers, all share the responsibility for student wellbeing. Such a goal requires coordinated approach underpinned by a student wellbeing policy. This chapter explores the common objections and potential risks to a school policy on student wellbeing. An overview of the evidence-based benefits of a student wellbeing policy then follows with the actions or recommendations a school, school system or nation(s) can take to develop a comprehensive student wellbeing policy.

3.1.1 Common Objections to a Student Wellbeing Policy

Traditionally, national education policy conversations have been about a country's competitiveness in terms of students' academic skills. Few countries have focused on student wellbeing as the driver for the development of educational policy.

© The Author(s) 2016   97
T. Noble and H. McGrath, *The PROSPER School Pathways for Student Wellbeing*,
SpringerBriefs in Well-Being and Quality of Life Research,
DOI 10.1007/978-3-319-21795-6_3

Traditional educational policies usually focus on the education of children and young people up to age 18 (or younger in countries with more limited formal education access) and the main educational debate has focused mostly on the access to, and the quality of a country's compulsory education system. Wealthier nations are somewhat fixated on data comparing the abilities of their nation's students on standardized academic tests, mostly in the areas of reading, writing, mathematics and scientific knowledge. The three data sets most commonly quoted are the International Mathematics and Science Study (TIMSS), the Programme for International Student Assessments (PISA) and the Progress in International Reading Literacy Study (PIRLS). PISA has been adopted as almost a global standard, and is now used in over 65 countries and economies (Breakspear 2012). Every three years, the release of PISA results stimulates a global discussion about school reform across many OECD and partner countries/economies. The 2012 Pearson report, 'The Learning Curve' used all three measures to create an overall index of cross-national educational attainment (Economist Intelligence Unit 2012). Approximately 150 countries do not currently take part in the studies; and it has been suggested that their failure to participate is because they would score far below the thresholds required for their inclusion to be statistically possible when standardising scores (Naumann 2005).

It is common for many countries to use these comparative indices to try to look for approaches used by the top-performing countries that appear to be associated with their success, especially educational policies for, and approaches to teacher training, national curriculum standards and annual standardised academic testing (Breakspear 2012). A focus on the impact of such policies on students' wellbeing is almost entirely missing. For many reasons this is problematic. For example there is convincing evidence that educational systems that incorporate high-stakes examinations combined with a culture of strong parental pressure can result in substantially reduced wellbeing for young people (Qin 2008). For example Yang and Shin (2008) found that the desire of Korean parents for their children to achieve highly in academic studies meant that their children's developmental needs for leisure, pleasure and sleep were often ignored, along with their psychological and emotional wellbeing needs. In fact according to the British Cohort Study the best predictor of a child becoming a satisfied and happy adult is not their academic achievement but their emotional health in childhood (Layard and Hagell 2015).

A focus on only academic outcomes as indicators of educational success is also an example of either/or thinking where educators see that it is either literacy or wellbeing; numeracy or wellbeing; rather than helping student to achieve both positive academic outcomes and enhanced wellbeing that help all students to flourish. A related objection is that a focus on student wellbeing requires a substantial budget that will take away resources from the academic curriculum. To illustrate that this does not need to be the case, each component of PROSPER in chap. 2 is supported by good teaching practices that do not require a substantial budget to drive change in student wellbeing and school system improvement.

3.1.2 Potential Risks Attached to a Student Wellbeing Policy

A school-based focus on student wellbeing is not a panacea that can solve all the challenges in education. Just focussing on improving student wellbeing does not mean that students' literacy and numeracy will automatically improve. The reality is of course that educators also need to explicitly teach literacy and numeracy skills to improve students' performance in these disciplines.

There is also a risk that some educators will take one well publicised research study at face value and assume that the practices advocated by that research will be appropriate for their students, school, district and country. The term 'gold standard' is often used to describe randomised control studies, a great many of which have been conducted with small samples of students under very controlled conditions that do not mirror the everyday reality of most classrooms and schools. Bauman et al. (1991) and Elias (2003) have noted that many programs are developed, trialled and maintained under almost-perfect conditions, with high levels of ongoing funding and professional support, high quality and well-trained staff, and high motivation. It is likely they will not successfully transfer to 'real school' conditions and schools can become somewhat discouraged when they do not perceive the same level of positive outcomes as were identified under the original ideal conditions.

It is very difficult and often prohibitively expensive to produce robust quantitative research data in authentic and naturalistic settings such as schools and many of the core variables being studied are often difficult to control across school settings. There is a high risk that a program is not continued once funding is withdrawn. Similarly, it can often be more difficult in education to establish causal relationships than it is in other professional practices. Also knowledge derived from older research studies may not be sufficiently up-to-date to meet the current needs of a school in the 21st century. Large scale quantitative research across a large number of schools may over-focus on the 'big picture' and, in doing so, miss some of the data from individual schools that may be most relevant to a specific school with a similar context.

3.1.3 Take an Evidence-Informed Approach to Student Wellbeing Policy and Practices

Schools are encouraged to take an evidence-informed approach that facilitates actions their school can take to put their student wellbeing policy into action. An evidence-informed approach means considering research that has been carried out in different countries, cultures, school systems and student populations, but also recognising that the research may need to be evaluated for it's appropriateness for an individual school's social and cultural context and educational system. Consideration should also be given to the factors that affect implementation of any initiative. Chap. 1 provides guidelines for choosing and implementing a student wellbeing program. Students involved in well-implemented social-emotional learning programs demonstrated academic gains that were twice as high as those students involved in poorly implemented programs (Durlak et al. 2011). The following Table 3.1 outlines five evidence-informed stages that contribute to the quality implementation of student wellbeing programs.

Table 3.1 Five Stages of Quality Implementation of Wellbeing Programs Based on Social-Emotional Learning

1. Selecting a Program
• Is the program evidence-informed?
• Does the program 'fit' with your school's vision and values?
• Can the program be customised to suit your school and address the needs of your students and school community without losing the program's core active ingredients?
• Is the program acceptable to your staff and school community?
• Are your leadership team and school administrators supportive?
2. Planning and preparing for implementation
• How can you gain the support of all staff involved in implementation?
• Is appropriate professional learning available for staff?
• Who will be in your program team and what are their responsibilities?
• How will the program team support the provision of resources that will help teachers in the program's implementation?
• Is your staff realistic about what the program can achieve?
• Will a member of the leadership team be able to coordinate the roll-out?
3. Implementation
• How will implementation be monitored so there is consistency of delivery and time allocation for the program?
• How will helpful feedback and support be regularly provided to teachers and how will any obstacles be identified and addressed?
• How will you encourage your staff to share their skills, knowledge and resources in relation to the program?
• How will you ensure reasonable fidelity to the program and consistency in time given to program delivery?
4. Sustaining the program
• How will you assess the impact of the program?
• How will you keep parents informed about the program to maintain their support?
• How will the program team refresh the program to maintain everyone's enthusiasm and commitment?
• How will the program team plan ahead for loss of key staff and the induction of new staff?
5. Improving the program
• How will you identify what's been working well and what can be improved?
• How will the staff be enabled to visit other schools that are implementing the program to explore and share ideas and resources?
• What additional professional learning and resources would add value?
• Adapted from Durlak, J.A. (2015) and McGrath & Noble (2011).

3.2 Developing Educational Policy for Student Wellbeing

Often educational policies in different countries have been developed in reaction to problems. For example the first Australian National Safe Schools Framework (NSSF) launched in 2004 was a response to widespread concerns about school bullying, harassment and violence. In collaboration with Erebus International we conducted a major evaluation and revision of this Framework in 2011. The vision of the new Framework is that schools are safe, supportive and respectful teaching and learning communities that promote student wellbeing. The Australian Government's Scoping Study on Approaches to Student Wellbeing (Noble et al. 2008) informed our development of the Safe Schools Framework (2011)—see Case Study page 107.

One of the goals of the Scoping Study on Approaches to Student Wellbeing, also commissioned by the Australian Government, was to explore the value of developing an overarching national framework/policy statement that encompassed a holistic approach to student wellbeing. This scoping study included a comprehensive literature review of the evidence-based school practices that promote student wellbeing and their academic engagement and a new definition of student wellbeing in consultation with national and international experts working in the field (see Chap. 1). The project also investigated the current national and international research and State/Territory government and non-government approaches to student wellbeing, in order to make recommendations about future Government directions in the area of student wellbeing. Feedback was sought from educators and key stakeholders in school and community agencies as well as school practitioners.

Policy development for enhancing student wellbeing emerged as a critical approach in the Scoping Study to the development of students' social, emotional and academic competence and a significant contribution to the ongoing battle to prevent youth depression, suicide, self harm, anti-social behaviour (including bullying and violence) and substance abuse. The methodology used in the Scoping Study to elicit the views of educators and leaders about the aspect of 'policy' included:

- Individual interviews with 40 Australian school leaders and administrators across different states, levels of schooling and educational systems. The 40 leading educators gave unanimous support for the development of a national framework or policy for student wellbeing (Noble et al. 2008).
- An online survey completed by 231 experienced teachers
- Two round table discussions with 32 teacher educators plus the use of keypad technology to enable them to respond anonymously to questions using a 1–5 Likert scale

The following section summarises the identified advantages of a national framework in student wellbeing. This summary draws on the Scoping Study research and on our research for a proposed revision of the Safe Schools Framework. A framework on student wellbeing is seen to have the following advantages:

3.2.1 Benefits of a National Policy on Student Wellbeing

A national policy on student wellbeing:

- *promotes an holistic education of the whole child*;
- *provides a common, shared national vision*, goals and agreed practices to develop sustained student wellbeing across all states and territories;
- *encourages a whole school approach* that engages all sectors of the school community in initiatives for student wellbeing to enhance student learning; a whole school approach also encourages sustainability of those initiatives
- *generates a common language* for teachers and the whole school community about the nature of student wellbeing and its enhancement in classrooms. This common language facilitates the opportunity for meaningful dialogue about student wellbeing within a school, across schools and across a nation or nations
- *connects wellbeing initiatives* enhances the capacity to 'join the dots' and link to other national student wellbeing initiatives and policies in education. The examples from the Australian education context are the Framework in Values Education, The Safe Schools Framework, Mental Health initiatives such as MindMatters (for secondary schools) and KidsMatter (for primary schools) and the National Schools Drug Education Plan.
- *creates economical benefits*: A traditional characteristic of educational policy is the concept of 'returns on investment'. An example of the costs-benefits of social-emotional learning programs was provided by a UK study that found that the costs of these programs were recouped in five years. A key driver of the calculation is the net savings in crime-related impacts of conduct problems that can be avoided plus the cost savings in health services after four years and the cost savings to the public sector after five years (Beecham 2014; Layard and Hagell 2015).
- *provides more educational equality*: Any new public policy in relation to education should also focus on educational equality if wellbeing is to be promoted. Access to education for girls varies significantly in different countries with girls far less likely to access education than boys in many less well resourced countries (Hausmann et al. 2009). Given the critical impact of maternal education on children's future educational achievement, health and wellbeing, limiting female access to education is very likely contributing to persistent inter-generational problems. Furthermore, where women have unequal access to the workplace—a usual consequence of unequal educational access—they are more likely to be in poverty, and have higher rates of depression, anxiety and suicide (Gaviria and Rondon 2010).
- *promotes a strengths-based perspective.*

A student wellbeing framework is also perceived to have the potential to change the dominant paradigm in many schools from a 'deficit perspective' to a 'positive, values and strengths-based pro-social perspective'. This shift in perspective is consistent with the positive education movement underpinned by the principles of positive psychology.

3.2.2 Policy Actions for Educational Policy Development for Student Wellbeing

The following actions could be adopted by any nation to facilitate their development of a student wellbeing policy.

(i) **Establish a platform for a framework policy for educating for student wellbeing**

- Seek common agreement and understanding of the key elements of a Framework Policy from the highest levels of decision-making in your country's Educational systems
- Ensure that the framework reflects the research evidence that confirms the link between education for student wellbeing and academic outcomes
- Be an advocate for the development of Professional Teaching Standards that describe what teachers need to know, understand and be able to do to support student social-emotional and academic learning
- Link the Framework to national and international Goals for Education and Skills for 21st century
- Seek agreement from stakeholders on the school pathways that underpin education for student wellbeing. Promote flexibility in the policy practices so that schools can adapt the pathways for their local social and cultural contexts.
- Focus on educating for student wellbeing from the early years prior to school, in school in both the primary and secondary school years, and post-school, including community options for lifelong learning.

(ii) **Collaboratively develop the framework with educational communities**

- Recognise and build on the work already undertaken on sustained student wellbeing in your educational communities at the local, national and international level
- Link to other current agendas in education and in youth development with common goals. These could include social-emotional learning, positive education/positive psychology, character education, values education, health/mental health promotion, restorative justice, positive behaviour support/positive behaviour for learning, mindfulness/meditation, bullying prevention, student-centred learning, service learning, values education, civics and citizenship, green schools, thinking skills and more.
- Develop a national/international monitoring and evaluation plan, including the development of performance measures to monitor the ongoing implementation of the Framework for Education for Sustained Student Wellbeing.
- Develop and disseminate support material and resources to assist schools to implement the Framework.

(iii) **Facilitate support for policy implementation in schools**

- *Implementation plan*: Develop a national/international implementation plan to monitor the ongoing implementation including support for school systems so they can provide support to schools. Indicate a suitable timeline for implementation that gives consideration to school planning cycles and funding support.
- *School Leadership*. Develop specific professional learning activities to engage school leaders in leading whole school wellbeing. Strengthening schools for sustainable student wellbeing will often involve significant school change and reform. Committed and inspiring leadership that models and articulates the school pathways for sustained student wellbeing can provide the vision, energy and focus over time to make a difference.
- Encourage the appointment of a *Leader, Director or Coordinator for student wellbeing* in each school. This person has the school leadership responsibility for the implementation of wellbeing initiatives/curriculum including monitoring progress of these initiatives across the whole school community.
- Adopt a *whole school approach* i.e. one that focuses on positive partnerships and assumes that all members of the school community (i.e. teachers, support staff, students and parents) share the same vision and values for student wellbeing and have a significant role/voice in promoting and sustaining a supportive school and connected culture. A whole-school approach also involves all areas of the school such as: policy and procedures, teaching practices, curriculum, code for positive school values and behaviour, positive behavioural support and the organisation and supervision of the physical and social environment of the school.
- Consider *choosing a whole-school social-emotional learning program* that will provide consistency across all school levels in teaching students the 21st century social-emotional skills for learning and for life. See Chap. 1 for guidelines on choosing and sustaining the implementation of SEL programs and in this chapter on adopting an evidence-informed approach. As noted in Chap. 1 many programs, usually target one age year level cohort in a school, and produce good results in the short term but these results are usually not sustained. This is not surprising given that the programs typically average 20 h (Durlak et al. 2011). A whole school program presented for one hour a week throughout a student's school life provides important opportunities for the key skills and understandings to be learned in age-appropriate ways and the repetition ensures a greater opportunity for deep 'habitual' learning (Layard and Hagell 2015; McGrath and Noble 2009).
- *Develop a professional learning plan* for all teachers tailored to the school's vision and agreed school practices for sustained student wellbeing. The professional learning plan may include:

- an initial communication strategy to schools and teachers regarding the nature and purpose of the student wellbeing educational policy and their role in, and responsibilities for, its implementation
- an ongoing professional learning plan to develop individual and collective teacher capacity for enhancing student wellbeing and learning
- guidelines for schools for building a supportive and connected school culture that enhances student learning and wellbeing.

- *Measure and document change.* Both quantitative and qualitative measures of improvement in student wellbeing and school climate provide important feedback to the whole school community. Government departments and school boards like to see quantitative evidence of improvement in key indicators of student wellbeing and school climate. As Stiglitz et al. (2009) noted, 'what we measure affects what we do' (p. 7).

  - *Whole School Measures:* The award-winning Safe Schools Hub provides a school audit tool for whole school wellbeing: Refer to: www.safeschoolshub.com.au
  - *Student Wellbeing Measures:* Given that student wellbeing is a multi-dimensional construct, then a multi-dimensional measure of student wellbeing is the most practical and useful approach for schools.

    (i) *PROSPER*: A measure of student wellbeing that incorporates each of the PROSPER components is currently under development. It is designed to provide feedback on each PROSPER component to help school leadership or teachers to identify strengths and gaps in individual or class student wellbeing.
    (ii) *The Well-Being Profiler* measures six empirically-derived dimensions of well-being: Psychological, Emotional and Strengths, Cognitive, Social, Physical, and Economic. The profiler has been developed by Dr. Tan Chyuan Chin in Centre for Positive Psychology Melbourne University. Schools can subscribe to the annual service and create an account. Schools will then have unlimited access to the survey and multiple surveys can be administered to students across the year. Schools will receive a tailored well-being profile report that contains useful information about the constructs measured. It is web-based, mobile-friendly, and compatible with Mac, PC and mobile devices (Android, iOS, Windows). http://wbprofiler.com
    (iii) *EPOCH scale* developed by Kern et al. (2014). It employs Seligman's PERMA model of wellbeing to develop the EPOCH scale for Adolescent Positive Functioning that yields a measure of Engagement, Perseverance, Optimism, Connectedness and Happiness.

(iv) *Warwick-Edinburgh Mental Wellbeing Scale* has also been adapted for adolescence. It is a 14 item scale that does not provide a multi-dimensional approach (Clarke et al. 2011).

(v) Penn University of Pennsylvania's authentic happiness website also provides a number of free wellbeing scales: www.authentichappiness.sas.upenn.edu including the adolescence VIA strengths scale or go to viacharacter.org

- *Involve Parents*—Provide advice to schools about how they can engage *Parents* and community-based organisations in the school's approaches to supporting education for student wellbeing, and
- *Teacher Education*—provide assistance to those engaged in the pre-service and postgraduate education of teachers to help them to better understand that student wellbeing is strongly linked to student learning and their responsibilities in this area.

3.2.3 Resourcing a Student Wellbeing Policy

Ideally your schools and district or nation's *Framework Policy for Educating for Student Wellbeing* will be available in multiple formats (electronic and paper) and readily accessible to schools. It is also well resourced, evidence-informed and includes many practical examples of good practice to guide schools in how to apply the Framework in their own school and classroom context. These resources may include whole school case studies plus resources and support materials that clearly demonstrate the inter-dependence of many school initiatives/pathways in ensuring sustained student wellbeing.

3.2.4 Background to Case Study: An Example of a Student Wellbeing Policy

The following case study provides an example of a student wellbeing framework. We were appointed by the Australian Government to conduct a review of the Safe schools Framework (Review of National Safe Schools Framework 2010) in collaboration with Erebus International which led to the revision of the Framework (2011).

The methodology for the revision included conducting a literature review and document analysis, consultation with 20 schools that represented good practice in student wellbeing (with a focus on student safety including cybersafety), and interviews with state/territory education representatives and key stakeholders to identify gaps in the original Safe Schools Framework (2003). The original framework was then redrafted and refined with further consultation with each of the above stakeholders on the revised draft.

A Case Study: The Australian Safe Schools Framework
A national school policy that focuses the attention of both Government ministers and school leadership to the crucial role of schools in promoting student wellbeing and resilience is illustrated by the Australian Government's (2011) National Safe Schools Framework; a framework endorsed by all State Ministers of Education and distributed to all schools in the nation.

This policy appears to be a world first in guiding all schools' curriculum and practices and highlights the Australian Government's endorsement of the important role of student wellbeing for learning and achievement. The vision of the Framework is to develop safe and supportive teaching and learning communities that promote student wellbeing.

'In a safe and supportive school, the risk from all types of harm is minimised, diversity is valued and all members of the school community feel respected and included and can be confident that they will receive support in the face of any threats to their safety or wellbeing' (p. 4)

The Framework identifies the following nine elements to assist schools in fulfilling this vision:

- Leadership commitment to a safe school
- Supportive and connected school culture (values and relationships)
- Policies and practices
- Professional learning (teacher education)
- Positive behaviour management approaches
- Student engagement, skill development and a safe school curriculum.
- A focus on student wellbeing and student ownership.
- Early intervention and targeted student and family support.
- Partnerships with families, community agencies and the justice system.

Schools are encouraged to conduct an online audit of their school's strengths and limitations based on these nine elements. The Framework provides examples of many evidence-based practices and resources for enhancing their school's capabilities for whole school, staff and student wellbeing and community-school partnerships.

The online 'safe schools hub' to support schools and teachers in their implementation of the Framework includes professional learning materials and case studies of schools that place a high priority on sustained student wellbeing. www.safeschoolshub.edu.au/

International e-Learning Award:
The Safe Schools Hub developed by Education Services Australia and supported by the Australian Government was awarded the prestigious International award for the best e-learning resource launched in 2014.

3.3   Conclusion

Education is central to happiness and wellbeing. It is the key to success in the development of social-emotional and academic learning and to success in life. The well-known African adage: *It takes a village to raise a child* reflects the critical importance of community partnerships for the wellbeing of children and young people. Schools are the most important community institution in any village, town or city. A school's partnership with the families in their school community and with local community groups and agencies is central to a school's effectiveness in providing an education for student wellbeing. School education is intrinsically dynamic and transformative. This book introduces a new conceptual framework called the PROSPER framework to first explain the multi-faceted seven elements that together contribute to wellbeing. These seven key elements are Positivity, Relationships, Outcomes, Strengths, Purpose, Engagement, and Resilience. Then the PROSPER framework is employed as an organiser for the evidence-based educational pathways that have been shown to help all students flourish. Case studies and research-to-practice examples help to illustrate how different school practitioners have implemented these pathways in their schools. Finally this publication overviews the benefits and policy actions of a student wellbeing policy for individual schools, and for school systems at the local, national and international levels.

References

Bauman, L. J., Stein, R. E., & Ireys, H. T. (1991). Reinventing fidelity: The transfer of social technology among settings. *American Journal of Community Psychology, 19*(4), 619–639.

Beecham, J. (2014). Annual research review: Child and adolescent mental health interventions: A review of progress in economic studies across different disorders. *Journal of Child Psychology and Psychiatry, 55*(6), 714–732.

Breakspear, S. (2012). *The policy impact of PISA: An exploration of the normative effects of international benchmarking in school system performance*, OECD Education Working Paper 71, OECD Publishing. http://dx.doi.org/10.1787/5k9fdfqffr28-en.

Briggs, F., & Hawkins, R. (1999). *Keeping ourselves safe*, SET special. New Zealand: NZCER.

Clarke, A., Friede, T., Putz, R., Ashdown, J., Martin, S., Blake, A., Adi, Y., Parkinson, J., Flynn, P., Platt, S., & Stewart-Brown, S. (2011). Warwick-Edinburgh Mental Well-being Scale (WEMWBS): Validated for teenage school students in England and Scotland. A mixed methods assessment. *BMC Public Health*, 11, 487. Retrieved from http://www.biomedcentral.com/1471-2458/11/487.

Durlak, J. A., Weissberg, R. P., Dymnicki, A. B., Taylor, R. D., & Schellinger, K. B. (2011), The impact of enhancing students' social and emotional learning: A meta-analysis of school-based universal interventions. *Child Development, 82*(1), 405–432.

Durlak, J.A. (2015). What everyone should know about implementation. In J.A. Durlak, C.E. Domitrovich, R.P. Weissberg & T.P. Gullotta (Eds.), *Handbook of social and emotional learning*. New York: The Guildford Press.

Elias, M. (2003). Academic and social-emotional learning. *International Academy of Education* I, 5–31.

Gaviria, S. L., & Rondon, M. B. (2010). Some considerations on women's mental health in Latin America and the Caribbean. *International Review of Psychiatry, 22*(4), 363–369.

Hammersley, M. (2005). The myth of research-based practice: The critical case of educational inquiry. *International Journal of Social Research Methodology, 8*(4), 317–330.

Hausmann, R., Tyson, L. D., Zahidi, S. (2009). *The global gender gap report.* World Economic Forum.

Kern, M.L., Waters, L.E., Adler, A., & White, M.A. (2014). A multidimensional approach to measuring well-being in students: Application of the PERMA framework. *The Journal of Positive Psychology.* Retrived from http://dx.doi.org/10.1080/17439760.2014.936962

Layard, R., & Hagell, A. (2015). Healthy Young Minds: Transforming the Mental Health of Children. In J.H. Helliwell, R. Layard & J. Sachs (Eds.), *World Happiness Report 2015.* New York: Sustainable Development Solutions Network. http://www.unsdsn.org/happiness

McGrath, H., & Noble, T. (2009). *The review and redevelopment of the national safe schools framework (NSSF).* Australian Government Department of Education, Employment and Workplace Relations.

McGrath, H., & Noble, T. (2011). *Bounce back! A wellbeing & resilience program. Lower primary K-2; middle primary: Yrs 3–4; upper primary/junior secondary:* Yrs 5-8. Melbourne: Pearson Education.

Naumann, J. (2005). TIMSS, PISA, PIRLS and low educational achievement in world society. *Prospects, 35*(2), 231–248.

Noble, T., McGrath, H. L., Roffey, S., & Rowling, L. (2008). *Scoping study into approaches to student wellbeing.* A report to the Department of Education, Employment and Workplace Relations.

Qin, D. B. (2008). Doing well vs feeling well: Understanding family dynamics and the psychological adjustment of Chinese immigrant adolescents. *Journal of Youth and Adolescence, 37,* 22–35.

Smith, P. K. (2001). Should we blame the bullies? *The Psychologist,* 14(2). (www.luckyduck.co.uk).

Stiglitz, J., Sen, A., Fitoussi, J.-P. (2009). *Report by the commission on the measurement of economic performance and social progress.* Retrieved from www.stiglitz-sen-fitoussi.fr/documents/rapport_anglais.pdf.

Yang, S., & Shin, C. S. (2008). Parental attitudes towards education: what matters for children's well-being? *Children and Youth Services Review, 30*(11), 1328–1335.